Optimizin
for the Pr

Optimizing Diabetes Care for the Practitioner

Irl B. Hirsch, MD

Professor of Medicine
Division of Metabolism, Endocrinology, and
  Nutrition
Medical Director, Diabetes Care Center
University of Washington Medical Center
Seattle, Washington

Dace L. Trence, MD, FACE

Assistant Professor
Division of Metabolism, Endocrinology, and
  Nutrition
Director, Diabetes Care Center
University of Washington Medical Center
Seattle, Washington

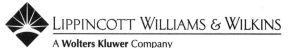

LIPPINCOTT WILLIAMS & WILKINS

A **Wolters Kluwer** Company

Philadelphia · Baltimore · New York · London
Buenos Aires · Hong Kong · Sydney · Tokyo

Acquisitions Editor: Brian Brown
Developmental Editor: Alyson Forbes
Production Editor: Emily Lerman
Manufacturing Manager: Ben Rivera
Cover Designer: Christine Jenny
Compositor: Lippincott Williams & Wilkins Desktop Division
Printer: RR Donnelley, Crawfordsville

Library of Congress Cataloging-in-Publication Data
0-7817-4161-0

Care has been taken to confirm the accuracy of the
information presented and to describe generally accepted
practices. However, the authors and publisher are not
responsible for errors or omissions or for any consequences from
application of the information in this book and make no
warranty, expressed or implied, with respect to the currency,
completeness, or accuracy of the contents of the publication.
Application of this information in a particular situation remains
the professional responsibility of the practitioner.

The authors and publisher have exerted every effort to
ensure that drug selection and dosage set forth in this text are
in accordance with current recommendations and practice at
the time of publication. However, in view of ongoing research,
changes in government regulations, and the constant flow of
information relating to drug therapy and drug reactions, the
reader is urged to check the package insert for each drug for
any change in indications and dosage and for added warnings
and precautions. This is particularly important when the
recommended agent is a new or infrequently employed drug.

Some drugs and medical devices presented in this publication
have Food and Drug Administration (FDA) clearance for limited
use in restricted research settings. It is the responsibility of the
health care provider to ascertain the FDA status of each drug or
device planned for use in their clinical practice.

10 9 8 7 6 5 4 3 2 1

This book is in the loving memory of
Gloria Hirsch and Fredis Trence

Contents

Preface ix
1. Defining the Issue: Why Focus on Diabetes
   Care?.. 1
   Age and Ethnicity 1
   Costs of Diabetes....................................... 3
   Avoidable Complications of Diabetes 3
   Future Predictions if No Intervention...... 4
2. Diagnosis... 5
   Criteria for Diagnosis 5
   Type 1 Diabetes.. 5
   Atypical Diabetes 8
   Pancreatic Diabetes.................................... 8
   Type 2 Diabetes.. 9
   Maturity-Onset Diabetes of the Young (MODY) 9
   Latent Autoimmune Diabetes of
       Adults and Type 1.5 Diabetes 10
   Type 3 Diabetes and Lipodystrophic
       Diabetes... 11
3. Getting Started in the Office. 13
   Self-Blood Glucose Monitoring 13
   Nutrition 15
   Physical Activity 16
   Hypoglycemia 17
   Ketones 17
   Goal Setting... 18
   Sick Day Management 18
4. Nonpharmacologic Therapies 20
   Medical Nutrition Therapy 20
   Exercise... 24
5. Pharmacologic Therapy 28
   Part 1: The Oral Agents.................. 28
       Insulin Secretagogues 30
       Insulin Sensitizers..................... 31
       α-Glucosidase Inhibitors 34
   Part 2: Insulin Therapy.................. 36
       Nomenclature 36
   Part 3: Supplements and Alternative
       Therapies for the Treatment of Diabetes . 46
       Select Micronutrients in Diabetes
           Management 46
       Products that May Treat the
           Complications of Diabetes 50
       Summary... 52
6. Acute Complications of Diabetes Mellitus 53
   Hyperglycemic Hyperosmolar Syndrome ... 53
   Diabetic Ketoacidosis 59

Diabetes Mellitus Is Associated with Many
Endocrinopathies.......................   63
Medications Resulting in Hyperglycemia ...   64
Severe Hypoglycemia   65
7. Microvascular and Neuropathic Complications   67
Mechanism of Microvascular Complications.   67
Diabetic Retinopathy...................   68
Diabetic Nephropathy...................   69
Neuropathy   73
8. Macrovascular Complications.............   77
Long-Term Mortality Comparisons........   77
Risk Factors for CVD in the Diabetic   79
9. Psychosocial Issues.....................   86
Barriers to Self-Care...................   86
Stages of Diabetes.....................   87
Behavioral Issues   90
Identification and Treatment of Common
Psychologic Disorders in Diabetes.......   90
Psychoeducational Intervention   92
10. Women and Diabetes....................   93
Adolescence   93
Reproductive Years   96
Menopause   100
11. Men and Diabetes......................   102
Puberty   102
Young Adulthood......................   102
Male Reproduction   103
12. Prevention of Diabetes   106
Lifestyle Modification   106
Medications...........................   107
Specific Behaviors   108
13. The Future of Diabetes Care..............   110
New Medications for the Treatment of
Hyperglycemia.......................   110
New Technologies for the Treatment of
Hyperglycemia.......................   111
New Technologies for Home Blood Glucose
Monitoring Data Management   111
New Medications for the Treatment of
Complications   112
Islet Cell Transplants   112

Appendix. Diabetes and You: Basic Information for
Patients Coping with Diabetes.................   113
Part   I: Diagnosis and Maintenance   115
Part II: Diet and Nutrition   141
Part III: Diabetes and Its Effect on
Your Body   157
Part IV: Diabetes and Your Well-Being.......   167
Subject Index   171

Preface

Diabetes mellitus is an old disease. Described vividly in the first century AD as a "melting down of flesh and limbs into urine" it was initially diagnosed through tasting the urine for sweetness, and treated with such approaches as watermelon seeds. By the beginning of the twentieth century, the diagnosis of type 1 diabetes was still a death sentence; for those who did not succumb to the disease, vascular complications were treated with raisins soaked in whiskey. By the late 1920s, it was clear that the introduction of insulin was not a cure. Despite many advances in the ensuing 80 years, we are now witnessing this disease double in incidence in just the past decade. The burden of the morbidity and mortality of diabetes continues to climb. With this lack of progress, why another book on diabetes?

Diabetes now accounts for roughly $0.25 of every Medicare dollar spent in healthcare. This fact alone is reason to focus on the prevention of the diabetes complications that the majority of these funds are required to treat. However, any attempt to calculate personal loss would reveal much more: the emotional costs of depression, the sense of loss of function, the difficulty in securing reasonably costly health or life insurance, even the ability to continue in specific professions or employment.

This book is focused on you, the primary provider of healthcare to the person with diabetes mellitus. It attempts to give you information that can rapidly be used to address typical day-to-day issues and standards of care. In addition, this book will provide an up-to-date review of how to handle the questions we all face every day while seeing patients, in addition to predicting the questions of the near future. Questions such as "is there a way to prevent diabetes, knowing I am at risk?" Or the common query asking "what about these supplements in treating my diabetes?" Questions about new technologies, new drugs, and even "cures" are common in every medical office in the United States. We have all learned that the Internet does not always provide the most accurate answers to these types of questions.

To quote from Dr. Christopher Suadek's 2002 Presidential Address at the American Diabetes Association Scientific Sessions:

"So I want, in closing, to offer each of you a challenge...Take it back to wherever you work and use it, improve on it, do it better, and come back for more. Because in this way each of

you, each of us, will contribute to the rising tide of diabetes research and care, until we have, in fact, found a cure."

Irl B. Hirsch, M.D.
Dace L. Trence, M.D.
February, 2003

Optimizing Diabetes Care for the Practitioner

Defining the Issue: Why Focus on Diabetes Care?

Diabetes is an epidemic occurring worldwide, and epidemics are rarely controlled unless their causes are identified or, at the very least, treatments are targeted to curb their devastating consequences. Among U.S. adults, diagnosed diabetes increased 49% between 1990 and 2000. Diabetes is now the sixth leading cause of death in the U.S., with over 200,000 Americans dying of diabetes-related complications yearly. Yet unrecognized by many people are that these complications of diabetes can be prevented. As an example, each year, 12,000 to 24,000 people become blind as a consequence of diabetic eye disease. Screening and subsequent targeted care could prevent 90% of diabetes-related blindness. However, only 60% of people with diabetes receive annual dilated pupil eye exams, so essential to recognizing the eyes at risk.

I. Age and ethnicity
A. National Health and Nutrition Examination Survey (NHANES) data from 1976 to 1980 showed a prevalence of diabetes of 8.9%. By 1988 to 1994, prevalence increased to 12.3% across all age populations.

    1. Currently, one in five adults over the age of 65 has diabetes mellitus.

    2. Among adults over the age of 20, African Americans are twice as likely as Caucasians to have diabetes, American Indians and Alaska Natives 2.6 times as likely.

    3. Type 2 diabetes affects 90% to 95% of people with diabetes, historically found typically in adults over age 40. With type 2 diabetes now increasingly found in children and teens, there is obvious concern as to future impact on health care and financial ability to meet these needs both globally as well as within the U.S. In the next 25 years, given current global trends, the estimated number of people with diabetes will increase from 150 to 300 million worldwide. Mexico's caseload will increase from under 5 million to 12 million, China's to 40 million, and India's will double from 30 to 60 million. Projections for the United States suggest an increase from 2000 to 2050 of 165% or an increased prevalence to 7.2%. According to the ongoing telephone survey of the Centers for Disease Control and Prevention Behavioral Risk Factor Surveillance System (BRFSS), the combined prevalence of diabetes and gestational diabetes increased from 4.9% in 1990 to 7.3% in 2000, an increase of 49%. Only 4 of the participating states reported a diabetes prevalence of ≥6% in 1990, but by 2000, that threshold was reached by 43 states. Very recent epidemiologic data suggest that the prevalence of diabetes in New York City alone has reached 8%.

a.   Type 2 diabetes is strongly associated with being overweight. BRFSS data on diabetes prevalence suggest that for every kilogram of increase in average self-reported weight, diabetes prevalence increases by 9%. Other studies have shown estimates of attributable risk of 27% for weight increases of 5 kg. An even more specific age-adjusted risk for the development of diabetes in women has been suggested by an increased waist-to-hip ratio, which adds to being overweight. In the Iowa Women's Study, women in the highest weight quintiles (as defined by body mass index) and with the highest waist-to-hip ratio had a relative risk of diabetes development of 29%. However, even women in the lowest body mass index quintile had an increased risk for diabetes if they also had a high waist-to-hip ratio.

b.   What biochemical criteria to use in defining diabetes has been increasingly more challenging to define, particularly when examining a point of transition from impaired glucose tolerance to frank diabetes. From the fasting plasma glucose level of over 140 mg/dL as proposed in 1979 to the current level of >125 mg/dL used since 1997, there remains considerable debate as to whether a fasting glucose level is really representative of a metabolic process that is associated with end-organ complication as compared to either postprandial glucose excursions or a combination of postprandial and A1c measurements reflecting glucose levels over time. It is anticipated that new criteria for diagnosis, already under discussion, will be proposed in the near future, which may further impact on the prevalence of diabetes and the socioeconomic burden this disease poses to the world.

II. Costs of diabetes

A. Average yearly health care cost in 1997 for a person with diabetes was $10,071 compared with $2,699 for a person without diabetes. Preventative treatment for cardiovascular disease per year (1997) was $3,120, but the postevent treatment rose to $9,385. Estimates in 2000 of lifetime medical costs for diabetes mellitus (types 1 and 2) were $233,000 versus $423,000 for women with cardiovascular disease; unfortunately, many women need treatment for both.

III. Avoidable complications of diabetes

A. Renal disease. About 38,000 people with diabetes develop end-stage renal failure yearly; 100,000 are actively treated for renal failure. Aggressive blood pressure and blood glucose control could reduce this kidney failure by 50%.

B. Amputations. About 82,000 people have diabetes-related leg and foot amputations each year. Eighty-five percent of these could be prevented through regular foot exams, including patient education on self-foot care with self-recognition of changes needing medical intervention.

C. Cardiovascular disease. Sixty-five percent of deaths in people with diabetes mellitus are related to heart disease and stroke. These deaths could be reduced by 30% through better blood pressure control, better glycemic control, and better lipid control. In U.S. 2000 dollars, based on the U.K. Prospective Diabetes Study, given current therapy trends, an A1c drift of 15% per year, in patients with 5 years of existing diabetes, estimated direct costs are approximately $47,240 per patient over 30 years, management of macrovascular disease accounting for 52% of cost, significantly more than nephropathy at 21%, neuropathy at 17%, and retinopathy at 10%.

D. Pregnancy complications. About 18,000 women with pre-existing diabetes deliver each year; an estimated 135,000 women are diagnosed with gestational diabetes. Screening for diabetes and diabetes care before and during pregnancy can reduce the risk of fetal wastage, congenital malformations, even the need for cesarean sections.

E. Infections. Yearly deaths in patients with diabetes mellitus from complications of flu or pneumonia are estimated at 10,000 to 30,000. People with diabetes are three times more likely to die of these complications than are people without diabetes. However, only 55% of people with diabetes receive an annual flu shot.

IV.   Future predictions if no intervention. In 1990, there was an average of 15.5 contacts with physicians per person with diabetes compared with 5.5 contacts per non-diabetic person. From 1981 to 1990, there was an increase of 50% in the number of visits with diabetes listed as a primary diagnosis. Diabetes was the second most frequently listed chronic disease prompting a visit to an office-based physician (hypertension was the first) in 1990. Clearly, the impact of diabetes cannot be ignored by any practicing physician, particularly family practitioners and general internists, who together account for almost 75% of these visits.

SELECTED READING

Boyle JP, Honeycutt AA, Narayan KM, et al. Projection of diabetes burden through 2050: impact of changing demography and disease prevalence in the U.S. *Diabetes Care* 2001;24: 1936–1940.

Caro JJ, Ward AJ, O'Brien JA. Lifetime costs of complications resulting from diabetes in the U.S. *Diabetes Care* 2002;25: 476–481.

Folsom AR, Kushi LH, Anderson KE, et al. Associations of general and abdominal obesity with multiple health outcomes in older women. *Arch Intern Med* 2000;160:2117–2128.

Harris MI, Flegal KM, Cowie CC, et al. Prevalence of diabetes, impaired fasting glucose, and impaired glucose tolerance in U.S. adults. The Third National Health and Nurition Examination Survey, 1988–1994. *Diabetes Care* 1998;21:518–524.

King H, Aubert RE, Herman WH. Global burden of diabetes, 1995–2025. *Diabetes Care* 1998;21:1414–1431.

Mokdad AH, Bowman BA, Ford ES, et al. The continuing epidemics of obesity and diabetes in the United States. *JAMA* 2001;286:1195–1200.

Rocchini AP. Childhood obesity and a diabetes epidemic. *N Engl J Med* 2002;346:854–855.

Diagnosis

Diabetes mellitus is a family of disorders of carbohydrate metabolism that are characterized by hyperglycemia, relative or absolute insulin deficiency, and the development of macrovascular, microvascular, and neuropathic complications. As we have learned more about the pathogenesis of the condition, diabetes classification has evolved accordingly. The latest classification by the American Diabetes Association (ADA) will likely be revised again.

I. Criteria for diagnosis. The most recent classification reports two major types of diabetes, with several less common forms. The diagnosis of diabetes is made based on one of three tests that must be confirmed on a subsequent day. These tests include a casual plasma glucose level of ≥200 mg/dL, a fasting plasma glucose level of ≥126 mg/dL, and a 75-g oral glucose tolerance test with a 2-hour value of ≥200 mg/dL. The 1997 conference also recognized intermediate levels of glucose intolerance. These include impaired fasting glucose, defined as a fasting plasma glucose level between 110 and 125 mg/dL, and impaired glucose tolerance, noted as a 75-g oral glucose tolerance test with a 2-hour level between 140 and 200 mg/dL. More recently, since the publication of the Diabetes Prevention Program, these two groups are now classified together as "prediabetes."

II. Type 1 diabetes. Type 1 diabetes is always associated with absolute insulin deficiency, and thus insulin is required for survival (Table 2-1). Type 1A diabetes (previously called insulin-dependent diabetes or juvenile-onset diabetes) results from a cellular-mediated autoimmune destruction of the β-cells of the pancreas.

A. Islet antibodies. Evidence of this autoimmunity can be found by the presence of one or more islet autoantibodies. None of these antibodies appear to play an etiologic role in β-cell destruction. However, they have developed a clinical utility in that two of these antibodies, islet cell antibodies (ICAs) and glutamic acid decarboxylase antibodies (GADAs), are now made available to clinicians by many commercial laboratories. In situa-

Table 2-1. Classification of diabetes mellitus

Type	Defect	Genetics	Therapeutics
Type 1	Autoimmune β-cell destruction	High-risk genetic markers confer increased susceptibility	Insulin
LADA	Autoimmune β-cell destruction (phenotypic type 1 diabetes)	High-risk genetic markers confer increased susceptibility	Insulin
Glucokinase MODY	Resetting of pancreatic glucose sensor	Mutation of glucokinase gene on chromosome 7	None
Transcription factor MODY	Insulin secretory defect	Mutation of hepatocyte nuclear factor genes and insulin promoter factor gene	Sulfonylurea or insulin
Type 2	Insulin resistance and relative insulin deficiency *not* due to autoimmune β-cell destruction	Likely polygenic	Sulfonylureas, metformin, α-glucosidase inhibitors, thiazolidinediones, insulin

Type 1.5	Insulin resistance (phenotypic type 2 diabetes) and insulin deficiency due to autoimmune β-cell destruction	Unknown	Unknown which therapies are best, but all available drugs likely work
Atypical diabetes	Nonautoimmune insulin deficiency and insulin resistance	Unknown, but autosomal dominant penetrance	Often initially requires insulin, but later can be well controlled on oral agents
Pancreatic diabetes	Insulin and glucagon deficiency	Variable—depends on etiology	Insulin
Lipodystrophic diabetes	Severe insulin resistance	Variable, based on whether congenital or acquired	Insulin sensitizers, insulin
Type 3 diabetes ("double diabetes")	Classic autoimmune β-cell destruction in childhood with later development of insulin resistance syndrome	Same high-risk genetic markers seen in type 1 diabetes in addition to family history of obesity and/or type 2 diabetes	Insulin ± insulin sensitizer

LADA, latent autoimmune diabetes of adults; MODY, mature-onset diabetes of the young.

tions where the etiology of the diabetes is not completely clear, the measurement of these antibodies may help to clarify the pathogenesis of the diabetes. Unfortunately, neither antibody is completely sensitive or specific, but as a general rule, the ICAs are better markers with children, whereas GADAs tend to have better results with adults. All of the antibodies, but particularly the ICAs, tend to diminish with time. The other two antibodies, insulin autoantibody and insulinoma-associated-2 autoantibodies, are still research tools but may become available for routine clinical use in the future. It should also be pointed out that serum insulin (or C-peptide) levels are not a good diagnostic tool for type 1 diabetes as early in the course of type 1 diabetes, especially latent autoimmune diabetes of adults (LADA; see page 6), endogenous insulin secretion will be present. Insulin secretion may be measurable for months and occasionally even years after diagnosis.

B. Associated conditions. Autoimmune destruction of the β-cells has multiple genetic predispositions and is also related to environmental factors that are still poorly defined. It should additionally be emphasized that the presence of obesity does not rule out the diagnosis of type 1A diabetes. Finally, individuals with type 1A diabetes are also prone to other autoimmune disorders such as Graves' disease, Hashimoto's thyroiditis, Addison's disease, celiac disease, selective immunoglobulin A deficiency, multiple sclerosis, juvenile rheumatoid arthritis, congenital rubella syndrome, and pernicious anemia.

III.   Atypical diabetes. Some forms of type 1 diabetes have no known etiologies (Table 2-1). These patients have permanent insulinopenia yet no islet autoantibodies. For example, only 47% of African Americans with new-onset type 1 diabetes are ICA positive, suggesting that a considerable proportion of African Americans with new-onset insulin-requiring diabetes do not have an autoimmune process. One possible diagnosis for this group would be atypical diabetes mellitus, a form of diabetes described in African Americans. Also called Flatbush diabetes, individuals with this diagnosis present with acute hyperglycemia with ketosis or ketoacidosis followed by a clinical course occasionally more typical of type 2 diabetes. It appears to be inherited as an autosomal dominant disorder.

IV.   Pancreatic diabetes. The other type of diabetes associated with severe insulin deficiency is termed pancreatic diabetes (Table 2-1). The etiology of the hyperglycemia is from diseases of the exocrine pancreas, such as pancreatitis, trauma or pancreatectomy, or neoplasia. Another common form of pancreatic diabetes is the diabetes associated with cystic fibrosis, termed cystic fibrosis–related diabetes. Individuals with pancreatic diabetes are usually insulin deficient but also very sensitive to insulin due to pancreatic glucagon deficiency.

V. Type 2 diabetes. Patients with type 2 diabetes have both insulin resistance and relative insulin deficiency (Table 2-1). Insulin therapy is not required for survival but is often necessary for the treatment of hyperglycemia. There are likely many different forms of this type of diabetes, and there is no autoimmune destruction of β-cells. Most people with type 2 diabetes have obesity-related insulin resistance. Although ketoacidosis seldom occurs spontaneously, it can be seen in association with other conditions that cause elevated counterregulatory hormones. Infection and myocardial infarction are particularly common etiologies of diabetic ketoacidosis, particularly in elderly patients.

A. Diagnostic clues. As with type 1 diabetes, serum insulin levels are not a good diagnostic tool for type 2 diabetes. Insulin levels are dependent on the blood glucose at the time of the blood draw, the antecedent glycemia, and the patient's insulin resistance. Insulin levels may be "low" if significant "glucose toxicity" has affected insulin secretion. Alternatively, serum insulin levels may be found to be "normal" or "high"; yet, in the context of hyperglycemia, the insulin level will always be *relatively insufficient*. Type 2 diabetes is often associated with a strong genetic predisposition, much more so than type 1 diabetes. Unfortunately, the genetics of type 2 diabetes are complex and not clearly defined. The major risk factors for type 2 diabetes include increased age, obesity, and lack of physical activity. It is also more common in individuals with hypertension or dyslipidemia, and its frequency is increased in Hispanics, African Americans, American Indians, and Asian Americans. It is also more common in women with a history of gestational diabetes or those women who delivered a baby with a birth weight over 9 lb.

VI. Maturity-onset diabetes of the young. Maturity-onset diabetes of the young (MODY) is a heterogeneous group of autosomal dominantly inherited disorders characterized by nonketotic diabetes, an onset usually in childhood or adolescence, and a primary defect in the function of the β-cells of the pancreas (Table 2-1). Clinically, some patients may have mild fasting hyperglycemia for many years, whereas others may have varying degrees of glucose intolerance before the onset of persistent fasting hyperglycemia. Occasionally, there may be rapid progression to overt hyperglycemia. According to recent estimates, MODY may account for 1% to 5% of all cases of diabetes in the United States and other industrialized countries. Currently, six different MODY mutations have been identified. However, these can be further classified as glucokinase MODY (mutations of the glucokinase gene) or transcription factor MODY (mutations in transcription factors).

A.   Glucokinase maturity-onset diabetes of the young. Glucokinase MODY, also known as MODY-2, is a mild, nonprogressive hyperglycemia caused by a re-setting of the pancreatic glucose sensor. It has been described in persons of all racial and ethnic groups. The mild fasting hyperglycemia (110 to 145 mg/dL) may often be recognized as early as at birth. Less than 50% of the carriers of this gene mutation have overt diabetes, and 50% of women carriers develop gestational diabetes. Diabetes-associated complications are rare in this form of MODY.

B.   Transcription factor maturity-onset diabetes of the young. All of the other MODY types currently identified are transcription factor MODY. As the defect is with insulin secretion, only insulin secretagogues and insulin are appropriate therapy. Identifying the type of MODY is difficult because few research labs do this testing. However, further information about exact identification may be found at *www.diabetesgenes.org*.

VII.   Latent autoimmune diabetes of adults and type 1.5 diabetes

A.   Latent autoimmune diabetes of adults. One of the first reports of an autoimmune process causing a slowly progressive form of type 1 diabetes in adults came in 1994. The authors showed that in 65 patients who presented with "adult-onset" diabetes, 19 required insulin therapy. These adult patients were, as a group, younger, with their onset of diabetes at an earlier age than the other 44 individuals. They also had lower postprandial C-peptide levels than the group not receiving insulin. Importantly, the frequency of GADAs was 74% in the group receiving insulin compared with 4% in those not. The conclusion from this report was that adults with newly diagnosed diabetes can have an autoimmune etiology leading to β-cell destruction and insulin deficiency. The pathogenesis of this form of diabetes is similar to that seen in classic type 1 diabetes of children, except that the β-cell destruction in the adults appears to be much more variable and usually much slower. Thus, the term *latent autoimmune diabetes of adults* (LADA) is used (Table 2-1).

B.   Type 1.5 diabetes. LADA is not a specific category in the ADA Committee Report for the Classification of Diabetes, but it is discussed. In one study, LADA subjects with a mean age of 54.5 years were found to have similar insulin resistance to that of an age-matched group of subjects with type 2 diabetes. The conclusion was that these overweight LADA patients (with a body mass index of 27.3 kg/m^2) share both the phenotypic characteristics and the insulin resistance seen in type 2 patients. Thus, some prefer the term type 1.5 diabetes (Table 2-1). Although used often in the literature, this latter term is not used in the most recent ADA classification. The literature is extremely confusing regarding how the terms LADA and type 1.5 diabetes are used. They are usually used interchangeably. What is agreed on is that all of these patients are positive to one of the islet antibodies.

   C.   Differentiating latent autoimmune diabetes of adults from type 1.5 diabetes. Until a new classification is developed, there will continue to be confusion with this group of patients. However, we tend to differentiate these two groups. Adults who develop diabetes, who are of normal weight (body mass index below 25.0 kg/m^2), and who are positive for one of the islet antibodies are generally considered to have LADA. Cases of overweight patients with a body mass index above 25 kg/m^2 who will likely be insulin resistant we tend to call type 1.5 diabetes. Phenotypically, the 1.5 group is indistinguishable from the classic patients with type 2 diabetes. Although there are many problems with this classification scheme, it assists in treatment strategies until definitive studies are completed.

      1.   Treatment. For patients with LADA, an autoimmune form of diabetes, the data regarding treatment are clear: Insulin therapy should be initiated. There are fewer data available for the best treatment for type 1.5 diabetes as defined here. One could make an argument for treating it with an insulin sensitizer and insulin secretagogue or insulin therapy soon after diagnosis as both an autoimmune attack on the β-cell and insulin resistance are present. The autoimmune attack, however, will lead to early insulin deficiency, and insulin therapy will usually be required earlier than in the patient with classic type 2 diabetes.

VIII.   Type 3 diabetes and lipodystrophic diabetes. To be complete, there are two final categories of diabetes that need to be mentioned. Type 3 diabetes, also called hybrid diabetes or double diabetes, is considered when a patient, usually a child, with classic type 1 diabetes develops insulin resistance later in life (Table 2-1). This is actually a common situation as it is estimated that 25% of the U.S. population is obese or has the syndrome of insulin resistance. We also see this in women who have type 1 diabetes and develop polycystic ovarian syndrome. Not surprisingly, these patients tend to respond well to insulin sensitizers, although there are few published data on this group. African Americans with type 3 diabetes have the typical autoimmunity seen in type 1 diabetes and thus need to be differentiated from the atypical diabetes described above. Lipodystrophic diabetes, associated with the lipodystrophies, is a syndrome of severe insulin resistance often with diabetes, hypertriglyceridemia, and fatty liver. It is characterized by selective but variable loss of fat tissue, with the degree of severity dependent on the amount of fat loss. Both familial and acquired lipodystrophies have been described, and these patients may require hundreds of units of insulin each day to control their diabetes.

SELECTED READING

Bergman RN, Finegood DR, Kahn SE. The evolution of beta-cell dysfunction and insulin resistance in type 2 diabetes. *Eur J Clin Invest* 2002;32(suppl 3):35–45.

Expert Committee on the Diagnosis and Classification of Diabetes Mellitus. Report of the Expert Committee on the Diagnosis and Classification of Diabetes Mellitus. *Diabetes Care* 2002;25:S5–S20.

Fajans SS, Bell GI, Polansky KS. Molecular mechanisms and clinical pathophysiology of maturity-onset diabetes of the youth. *N Engl J Med* 2001;345:971–980.

Garg A. Lipodystrophies. *Am J Med* 2000;108:143–152.

Libman IM, Pietropaolo M, Trucco M, et al. Islet cell autoimmunity in white and black children and adolescents with IDDM. *Diabetes Care* 1998;21:1824–1827.

Liu E, Eisenbarth GS. Type 1A diabetes mellitus-associated autoimmunity. *Endocrinol Metab Clin North Am* 2002;31: 391–410.

Palmer JP. Beta cell rest and recovery: does it bring patients with latent autoimmune diabetes in adults to euglycemia? *Ann NY Acad Sci* 2002;958:89–98.

Palmer JP, Hirsch IB. What's in a name? LADA vs type 1.5 vs adult-onset type 1 diabetes. *Diabetes Care* 2003;26:536–538.

Getting Started in the Office

Initial management decisions should be based on the metabolic stability of the patient with newly diagnosed diabetes. Increasingly common is the diagnosis of diabetes in medical evaluation for a medical concern other than the classic symptom presentation of polyuria, polydipsia, and weight loss. Fatigue, nocturia, and leg cramping are not infrequently reported symptoms that bring the patient in, seeking evaluation for suspected other etiology than diabetes mellitus. Often the diagnosis is made from laboratory tests obtained to screen for etiology of presenting concerns. The initial approach is to implement what is frequently termed survival skills teaching, as the patient deals with the emotional aspects of hearing a diagnosis that is many times associated with a devastating outcome in a family member or friend. Too often there is an attempt to provide education on issues such as the pathophysiology of diabetes before the patient has a chance to deal with the acuteness of hearing the diagnosis, in addition to not feeling well. Focus should be placed on engaging the patient in obtaining data that will help in the decision process as to optimal therapy. Providing information on all the nuances of self-management of diabetes should be in stages, as the patient is ready for it.

I. Self-blood glucose monitoring. Glucose monitoring is key to decision making, from the aspect of both the health care provider as well as the patient. Fingerstick glucose determinations can be made quickly, with chemical reaction for a reading taking as short a time as 5 seconds, with as little volume as 0.03 μL of blood (an amount similar to the area of the head of a small pin), on many of the newer-generation glucose meters. Alternative sites to fingertips can be used if checking premeal glucose levels or when glucose levels are not suspected to be widely fluctuating. These alternate sites include the forearm (the inner forearm is a better site to more easily obtain blood), thigh, and calf. Urine glucose determinations should be avoided, as the renal threshold for glycosuria is 180 mg/dL and commonly reflects blood glucose well as it was typically over 3 hours previously. Self-blood glucose monitoring (SBGM) discomfort can be minimized by lancet-holding devices that allow for adjustment of the depth of needle puncture, instructing the patient to start glucose self-monitoring on the tips of the fourth and fifth digits (less sensitive than others), and instructing that the lancet be directed to between the tip and the margins of the digit.

A.   Disadvantages of SBGM are few other than expense. There is the potential of infection, nerve damage, and discomfort despite the above guidelines, but cost can be a barrier particularly if insurance coverage is not available. Initiating a twice-daily regimen, alternating between prebreakfast and predinner with prelunch and bedtime, can rapidly yield a pattern of glucose levels that allow decision making regarding further therapeutic intervention in just a few days yet can minimize the cost.

B.   Optimal frequency of SBGM will be determined by the patient's metabolic stability, the therapeutic intervention planned, the type of diabetes, and the patient's willingness. The patient with typical type 2 diabetes will initially benefit from at least twice-daily checking, but more may be needed if dietary choice is to be evaluated in the treatment plan, if the effects of physical activity are to be reviewed, and certainly if initiated oral medication begins to take effect. If insulin is initiated, then, depending on the protocol chosen, four-times-daily checking will be preferable, until the effect of dose and type of insulin can be evaluated and the patient has reached target glycemic control. The patient with type 1 diabetes will need minimally premeal and bedtime glucose evaluations, as metabolic instability is typically part of the initial presentation.

   1.   Even the patient with glucose levels that are <200 mg/dL can benefit from glucose monitoring as a tool for decision making. Medication used alone should not be a criterion for encouraging the ongoing use of SBGM. Dietary choices made can be evaluated by SBGM at 1 to 2 hours after a meal or snack, giving patients immediate feedback as to whether their choice of food or portion size was one that allowed for metabolic stability or facilitated a large glucose rise. The effect of physical activity or exercise can be another reason to encourage SBGM both before as well as after exercise to evaluate glucose effects.

   2.   Limitations in sight, which might be even more apparent in the newly diabetic patient, can affect focusing ability and therefore the ability to use a glucose meter. Magnifying lenses can be placed over digital print to enhance clarity; some meters give an auditory cue notifying the patient of the adequacy of the blood sample for strip processing. Meters for sight-limited individuals are available, with auditory cues validating the adequacy of the blood sample and informing of the actual glucose result. For patients with impaired dexterity, the appropriate size of the strip to be used should be determined by observing the patient through an SBGM process.

3. The glucose watch can be considered for persons who wish to be able to check their glucose frequently without consistently doing a finger stick; however, calibration still requires finger-stick glucose determination. Most limiting to this approach is the current expense of both the watch device and the membrane required for skin-to-watch contact for glucose determinations. Even continuous glucose sensors with capacity for 72-hour glucose determinations could be considered in occasional newly diagnosed patients for initial glucose determinations, although this tool also requires initialization as well as ongoing calibration through SBGM.

4. Patients should be instructed to check their glucose in special situations. These include illness; changes in well-being, scheduled physical activity, work, mealtimes, or caloric intake; or when questioning symptoms of possible hypoglycemia.

II. Nutrition. It is the rare patient who will not ask for some information regarding dietary changes at the time of initial diagnosis. Medical nutrition therapy has changed dramatically in the approach to diabetes, with liberalization of recommendations from the early "starvation diet" approach. The initial recommendation should be to focus on a healthy overall food intake, with a goal of weight management and an emphasis on beginning to read food labels to review carbohydrate intake. Although the specifics of dietary adjustments are not part of survival skills management, the patient can often benefit from a dietary recall or keeping a food diary that then allows the ability to correlate glycemic response to food and portion of food chosen. Web sites such as *www.calorieking.com* can be helpful to the patient looking at brand-name foods as well nonlabeled foods in the beginning to learn food content.

A. Initial recommendation should be to decrease concentrated carbohydrate intake. Frequently, polydipsia has been treated with regular carbonated beverages, only adding to the glycemic load. Diet pop or soda, according to patient preference, should be substituted for regular pop or soda, but as many newly diagnosed individuals are dehydrated, water intake should be encouraged. Patients should be advised that coffee and tea are diuretic, and alcohol should be avoïded until hyperglycemia is controlled.

B. Becoming aware of carbohydrate content in chosen foods is a skill that takes time to develop, and creating a carbohydrate budget can be helpful, until the patient can be seen by a registered nutritionist or diabetes educator and an individualized plan formulated. Taking basal calorie needs as 10 to 12 kcal/lb of desirable weight, adding 30% extra if sedentary, 50% extra if moderately active, and 100% if strenuously active, an initial recommendation of approximately 60% of daily calories from carbohydrate can be suggested. Often a bit bewildering to patients, this can be simplified to suggesting a targeted level of 45 to 60 g of carbohydrate per meal, with encouragement to begin looking at food product labels for the carbohydrate content, until an individualized plan specific to the patient's needs can be formulated.

C. Weight management is often an additional focus, particularly in the patient with type 2 diabetes. Creating an awareness of sizes of food portions can be a good starting point: 3 to 4 oz being the size of a deck of playing cards or the size of a computer mouse, 1 oz the size of a thumb. For liquids, can label contents can be helpful, or comparisons can be made to a small cup of coffee as 8 oz.

III.   Physical activity. Exercise is an important component of initial survival skills teaching. The opportunity to encourage an increase in physical activity should not be missed, although the newly diagnosed person with diabetes needs to be cautioned regarding the potential effect of aggressive exercise to paradoxically further increase blood glucose. Generally, a blood glucose level of ≤240 mg/dL should be used as a guide below which glucose will typically decrease with activity. Any aggressive physical activity should be avoided until the patient has had a cardiovascular disease risk assessment and evaluation. Additionally, any patient with active proliferative retinopathy should avoid exercise that increases intra-abdominal pressure or results in Valsalva-like maneuvers (lifting weights). Patients with peripheral neuropathy should avoid running due to risk for pedal trauma and injury. However, starting a walking program, encouraging selection of an enjoyable activity to the patient such as swimming or biking, or even using a lunchtime break to walk around the place of employment can foster glycemic improvement because of increased peripheral insulin sensitivity and consequent glucose disposal. An activity diary coupled with glucose determinations can be helpful to target additional treatment interventions. The effect of exercise can persist for up to 12 hours, with hypoglycemia often being a high risk, particularly after strenuous exercise.

IV.   Hypoglycemia. As important as controlling hyperglycemia are the awareness and recognition of the symptoms of hypoglycemia. As the patient modifies diet and activity coupled with often-indicated initial pharmacologic intervention, the symptoms and treatment of hypoglycemia require that it be included in survival skills teaching. Symptoms include diaphoresis, shakiness, palpitations, headache, intense sense of hunger, and confusion. Typically, the same symptoms will be appreciated by the person with recurrent episodes, so that the symptoms should become the heralding sign needing prompt attention. Initially, patients should be encouraged to check their glucose if there is any question of change of well-being. The level at which hypoglycemic symptoms occur will vary according to the glycemic level at which patients are accustomed to being, their general health, age, sex, and even the duration of diabetes. A level below 60 mg/dL is generally an accepted level below which the risk of significant cognitive impairment is present. However, with increasing age and co-morbidities, this cut-off should be considered at much higher levels such as 80 mg/dL. The accepted definition of severe hypoglycemia is that requiring assistance to treat, patients not being able to treat themselves. Mild hypoglycemia and that during the night might require less carbohydrate than hypoglycemia during the daytime due to skipped meals or strenuous exercise.

Treatment with concentrated carbohydrate sources of 10 to 30 g should be used for moderate hypoglycemia. Options include 2 to 3 glucose tabs (5 g each), one-third to one-half a tube of 30 g of glucose gel, 4 to 6 oz of orange juice, 4 to 6 oz of nondiet cola, and one-fourth to one-third a cup of raisins. If the glucose does not respond in 15 minutes or symptoms persist, treatment should be repeated. For severe hypoglycemia, twice the initial intake should be used, and then both should be followed by a protein- or fat-containing meal such as half a meat sandwich or bowl of cold cereal with milk. If the patient cannot ingest glucose orally, intramuscular or subcutaneous glucagon will be needed. These are issues more often needing attention when pharmacologic intervention is started.

V.   Ketones. Ketone checking should be included in survival skills instruction. Although the vast majority of patients with type 2 diabetes will not need to continue this skill, it is important to learn how to check urine ketones at initial diagnosis, as an aid to managing sick days in the future. Patients should be instructed that ketones signify a change in body metabolism—which can occur with glucose levels above 240 mg/dL; this is why their glucose meter may suggest ketones be checked above this glycemic threshold. Ketoacidosis symptoms may be indistinguishable from gastroenteritis symptoms, with a moderate to strong presence being the defining differential.

VI. Goal setting. Goal setting is critical to guide both the patient and the provider in planning and evaluating therapy. Specific goals such as glucose levels should be initial targets and secondarily long-term targets. The patient who presents with a glucose level of 300 mg/dL might have a targeted initial glycemic goal set of all values <200 mg/dL, but the eventual goal might be <150 mg/dL. Patients need to hear what is considered ideal glycemic control to establish a treatment plan; if glycemic goals are not reached with one approach, then a working relationship has been established to proceed to the next intervention. Hemoglobin A1c (A1c) values need to be discussed, with definitions provided and targets that are safe and yet ultimately provide less risk of long-term complications. For the patient who presents with an initial A1c of 10%, the next goal might be an A1c level in the single digits, such as in the 8 or 9 range; the eventual goal is in the 6.0 range. An A1c determination should be obtained early in the initial treatment of diabetes.

Paramount is the need to discuss symptom control first, as even the patient without polyuria or polydipsia will typically report an improvement in energy with improvement in glycemic control.

VII. Sick day management. Sick day management should be reviewed as part of survival skills teaching. When illness occurs, patients should be instructed in the need to check glucose every 2 to 4 hours and, if the patient has type 1 diabetes, to check urine for ketones every 4 hours if glucose is above 240 mg/dL. If patients are on insulin, they will need to be instructed in the use of supplemental doses of either short-acting or rapid analog insulin (typically 0.1 to 0.3 U/kg every 2 to 4 hours). Need to discontinue metformin, if this is being used, should be discussed, but other glycemic control medications should be continued. Many patients feel that if they are not eating, glycemic control medications should be discontinued, so continued use of medication should be specifically reviewed. Fluid intake is essential to prevent dehydration. If not possible orally, due to nausea or emesis, then intravenous replacement should be started. Oral intake of fluids such as popsicles, clear soups, and flat nondiet soda is recommended to provide some electrolyte and carbohydrate replacement. Failure to improve, inability to keep fluids down, increasing lethargy, or inability to continue SBGM should be reasons to direct the patient to the emergency room or urgent care center for evaluation for admission for treatment.

SELECTED READING

Glascow RE, Toobert DJ, Hampson SE. Effects of a brief office-based intervention to facilitate diabetes dietary self-management. *Diabetes Care* 1996;19:835–842.

Nathan DM. Monitoring diabetes mellitus. In: Leibovitz H, ed. *Therapy for diabetes mellitus and related disorders,* 3rd ed. Alexandria, VA: American Diabetes Association, 1998;109–117.

Norris SL, Engelgau MM, Venkat Narayan KM. Effectiveness of self-management training in type 2 diabetes. *Diabetes Care* 2001;24:561–587.

Norris SL, Lau J, Smith SJ, et al. Self-management education for adults with type 2 diabetes. *Diabetes Care* 2002;25:1159–1171.

Nonpharmacologic Therapies

I. Medical nutrition therapy

A. Introduction. People with diabetes and health professionals recognize nutrition therapy as one of the most challenging aspects of diabetes care. A current American Diabetes Association (ADA) or diabetes diet can only be defined as a dietary prescription based on desired health outcomes. Appropriate self-management training must be goal directed and requires an individualized approach.

B. Goals of therapy

1. Attain and maintain optimal metabolic outcomes including:

    a. Blood glucose levels in the normal range or as close to normal as is safely possible to prevent or reduce the complications of diabetes.

    b. A lipid profile that reduces the risk of macrovascular disease.

    c. Blood pressure levels that reduce the risk for vascular disease.

2. Prevent and treat the chronic complications of diabetes.

3. Improve health through healthy food choices and physical activity.

4. Address individual nutrition needs, taking into consideration personal and cultural preferences and lifestyle while respecting the individual's wishes and willingness to change.

C. Principles of therapy

1. Type 1 diabetes. Use self-monitoring of blood glucose to adjust food intake and insulin dose.

    a. For youths with type 1 diabetes, provide adequate energy to ensure normal growth and development.

2. Type 2 diabetes. If obese, restrict calories for moderate weight loss; the focus should be on a decrease of fat intake, improved food choices, and spacing meals throughout the day.

3. For pregnant and lactating women, provide adequate energy and nutrients needed for optimal outcomes.

4. **For older adults,** provide for the nutritional and psychosocial needs of an aging individual.

5. **For individuals at risk for diabetes,** decrease risk by encouraging physical activity and promoting food choices that facilitate moderate weight loss or at least prevent weight gain.

D. **Carbohydrates and diabetes.** There has been much confusion about what types of carbohydrates cause the greatest glycemic rise. It is now clear that the total amount of carbohydrate in meals and snacks will be more important than the source or the type. In fact, sucrose does not increase glycemia to a greater extent than isocaloric amounts of starch- and sucrose-containing foods. Therefore, sucrose does not need to be restricted in people with diabetes, but these foods need to become part of the usual meal plan or covered with insulin or glucose-lowering medication. Ideally, individuals receiving intensive insulin therapy should adjust their premeal insulin dose based on the carbohydrate content of meals. "Carbohydrate counting" has become quite popular, so that a predetermined amount of insulin is provided for a given amount of carbohydrate. For example, a typical carbohydrate ratio for a person with type 1 diabetes would be 1 U of prandial insulin (e.g., insulin lispro or aspart) for every 15 g of carbohydrate. The more insulin-resistant type 2 patient might start at 1 U of insulin for every 10 g of carbohydrate. Very insulin-resistant patients may need much more aggressive ratios. An example would be as follows: A 50-year-old man with type 2 diabetes and a carbohydrate ratio of 1 U/10 g of carbohydrate has a cup of corn flakes (25 g), 1 cup of 2% milk (15 g), and 1 cup of unsweetened orange juice (25 g). This calculates to 65 g of carbohydrate and, based on the ratio, will require 6.5 U of insulin. Although we usually round up for this, insulin pens that can deliver insulin in 0.5-U increments are now available. This is particularly helpful for people who are extremely insulin sensitive. There are numerous outstanding books with tables of carbohydrate content, and there are also computer programs that allow downloads of carbohydrate contents to personal digital assistants. There are also several web sites available that deal solely with the carbohydrate content of various foods, including those from fast-food restaurants. One of these web sites is *www.calorieking.com*, which also has a "diabetes tracker" on the site.

1. **Type 1 diabetes.** There is a strong relationship between the premeal insulin dose and the postprandial response. Therefore, the premeal insulin dose should be adjusted for the content of the meal,

which is usually accomplished by the carbohydrate-counting method. For individuals receiving a fixed dose of mealtime insulin, day-to-day consistency in the amount of carbohydrate is important. Whichever strategy is utilized, this therapy requires a nutritionist for optimum efficacy.

2.   Type 2 diabetes. On a weight maintenance diet, replacing carbohydrate with monounsaturated fat reduces postprandial glycemia and triglyceride levels. The concern is that this increase in fat could promote weight gain. Thus, the contributions of carbohydrate and monounsaturated fat need to be individualized with the assistance of a nutritionist knowledgeable about this topic.

E.   Protein intake and diabetes. Studies have found that in persons with controlled type 2 diabetes, ingested protein does not increase plasma glucose concentrations, although protein is as potent a stimulant of insulin secretion as carbohydrate. Current ADA recommendations suggest that a usual protein intake of 15% to 20% of total daily energy is appropriate, assuming normal renal function. Long-term effects of high-protein, low-carbohydrate diets are unknown. These diets clearly do produce short-term weight loss and improved glycemia, but long-term outcomes have not been published. Furthermore, the low-density lipoprotein (LDL)–cholesterol levels increase with these diets, and the effect of this is a concern.

F.   Dietary fats and diabetes. Less than 10% of energy intake should be derived from saturated fats. Some individuals may benefit from lowering saturated fat intake to <7% of energy intake. Dietary cholesterol intake should be <300 mg per day. Some individuals may benefit from lowering dietary cholesterol to <200 mg per day. To lower LDL-cholesterol, energy derived from saturated fat can be reduced if weight loss is desirable or replaced with either carbohydrate or monounsaturated fat when weight loss is not a goal. Reduced-fat diets when maintained over the long term contribute to modest loss of weight and improvement in dyslipidemia.

G.   Ethnic groups. One of the traditional mistakes made in teaching the principles of meal plans for people with diabetes is that the cultural aspects of the types of food eaten are not addressed. For a Hispanic patient, for example, one needs to be sensitive about how to incorporate the foods normally eaten at home into the meal plan. This may require a change in the type of insulin used or perhaps the need to take insulin only for certain meals. Similarly, for Asian patients, for whom rice is a main part of the diet, we have found the insulin analogs to be a valuable tool to assist in controlling the post-prandial rise that often occurs. These are just examples of the important point that, when discussing food, we need to remember that our patients may have very different food habits that will not be able to change because of the diagnosis of diabetes.

H. Nonpharmacologic treatment of obesity. This can be very difficult as it depends on patient readiness: the need to make a long-term lifestyle commitment for success. The provider must appreciate that not all patients are willing or able to make such commitments, and the patient has the right to decline treatment.

1. Structured programs that emphasize lifestyle changes, including education, reduced fat (<30% of daily energy) and energy intake, regular physical activity, and regular participant contact, can produce long-term weight loss on the order of 5% to 7% of starting weight. Standard weight reduction diets, when used alone, are unlikely to produce long-term weight loss. Structured intensive lifestyle programs are necessary.

2. Weight loss. A prescription for weight loss must include a calorie deficit. Eating 500 to 1,000 cal per day less than usual or less than maintenance calorie needs should result in a weight loss of 1 to 2 lb per week (Table 4-1). The minimum recommended calorie level is 1,200 for women and 1,500 for men to ensure the diet is nutritionally adequate in vitamins and nutrients. To assist in weight loss and maintenance, increased physical activity is recommended.

I. Pharmacologic treatment of obesity. These agents are a useful adjunct to, but not a substitute for, changes in food intake and physical activity. Pharmaco-

Table 4-1. Estimating calorie needs of adults

Basal calories
    10–12 kcal/lb desirable body weight
    20–25 kcal/kg desirable body weight
Add calories for activity
    If sedentary, additional 30% calories
    If moderately active, additional 50% calories
    If strenuously active, additional 100% calories
Adjustments
    Add 300 kcal/d during pregnancy
    Add 500 kcal/d during lactation
    Subtract 500 kcal/d to lose 1 lb/wk

logic intervention is recommended for use in people with diabetes with a body mass index (BMI) above 27 kg/m^2. For those with no co-morbid conditions, they are appropriate only if the BMI is above 30 kg/m^2.

    1.   Sibutramine (Meridia). Although this agent needs to be used with caution in patients with diabetes owing to problems with tachycardia and hypertension, it can be used safely in selected patients. Start at 10 mg per day, and titrate to 15 mg per day if weight loss is inadequate (<4 lb in the first 4 weeks); it can be taken with or without food, and no vitamin supplements are required. In a study of 1,047 patients, the 15-mg dose produced a weight loss of 7 kg at 24 weeks. At 1 year, 3% of subjects maintained a 10% loss from initial weight. Most common side effects are headache (30%), dry mouth (17%), anorexia (13%), constipation (12%), and insomnia (11%). It substantially increases blood pressure and heart rate in some patients; thus, regular monitoring is required. It should not be used in patients with a history of coronary artery disease, arrhythmia, congestive heart failure, or stroke.

    2.   Orlistat (Xenical). This agent acts locally to inhibit gastrointestinal lipases, blocking the absorption of approximately 30% of dietary fat. Absorption of carbohydrates and proteins is not affected. In one 2-year study with 133 subjects in the orlistat group and 123 in the placebo group, approximately 25% of subjects receiving active drug maintained a 10% reduction in body weight compared with 6.5% receiving placebo. Over 45% of orlistat-treated subjects reduced body weight by >5% compared with 24% of placebo-treated patients. The greater the weight loss, the greater the LDL-cholesterol reduction (14.5% reduction if >10% weight loss). In patients with type 2 diabetes on sulfonylureas, more patients on orlistat compared with placebo were required to discontinue their sulfonylureas, and hemoglobin A1c levels were improved with the orlistat group. As orlistat can inhibit the absorption of fat-soluble vitamins, it is suggested that patients receiving orlistat receive a multivitamin supplement 2 hours before or after the ingestion of the drug. The most common side effects are oily spotting, flatus with discharge, fecal urgency, fatty/oily stool, oily evacuation, increased defecation, and fecal incontinence.

II.   Exercise

A.   Introduction. Regular exercise is recommended as an important component of therapy for all people with diabetes. In 2002 the National Academies' Institute of Medicine recommended 60 minutes of exercise per day, twice as much as previous recommendations.

B. Benefits. For some patients with type 2 diabetes, a regular exercise program may be the main treatment of the diabetes. Physical training results in improved insulin sensitivity as noted by decreased fasting and postprandial insulin levels. Both oral agent and insulin doses may need to be decreased in people with type 2 diabetes who begin an exercise program. In those with type 1 diabetes, insulin requirements will be decreased with exercise. Other nonglycemic benefits include improved lipid levels (especially triglyceride levels) and improvement in mild or moderate hypertension. As noted above, regular exercise clearly helps with weight loss. Finally, an exercise program will improve cardiovascular fitness and improve sense of well-being and quality of life.

C. Pre-exercise evaluation. Prior to exercise, a thorough evaluation should carefully screen for the presence of macro- and microvascular complications.

1. Cardiovascular disease. A graded exercise test may be helpful if a patient, about to embark on a moderate- to high-intensity exercise program, is at high risk for underlying cardiovascular disease, based on one of the following:

a. Age > 35 years
b. Type 2 diabetes of >10 years' duration
c. Type 1 diabetes of >15 years' duration
d. Presence of any other risk factors for coronary artery disease
e. Presence of microvascular disease
f. Peripheral vascular disease
g. Autonomic neuropathy

In patients with nonspecific electrocardiogram changes, a radionuclide stress test should be considered. In those planning to participate in low-intensity forms of exercise (<60% of maximal heart rate) such as walking, clinical judgment is required to decide if an exercise stress test is required.

2. Diabetic retinopathy. Yearly dilated eye exams should be performed as per ADA recommendations because active, strenuous activity may precipitate vitreous hemorrhage.

3. Diabetic nephropathy. The presence of proteinuria per se is not a contraindication to vigorous physical activity. However, proteinuria is a strong independent risk factor for coronary artery disease, and thus these individuals should also have exercise stress testing.

4. Peripheral neuropathy. The main concern here is that the loss of protective sensation makes repetitive exercise on insensate feet a high risk for ulceration. The inability to detect sensation using the 5.07 (10-g) monofilament is indicative of the loss of protective sensation. These high-risk patients require cushioned shoes and frequent self-exams for preulcer areas that would require treatment.

5. Autonomic neuropathy. Patients with cardiac autonomic neuropathy have a heart rate above 100 beats/min (parasympathetic dysfunction) or orthostasis (sympathetic dysfunction). Sudden death has been attributed to cardiac autonomic dysfunction. Therefore, resting or stress thallium myocardial scintigraphy is an appropriate test in these individuals.

D. Warm-up and cool-down periods. A warm-up period should consist of 5 to 10 minutes of aerobic activity at a low-intensity level. Muscles should then be gently stretched for 5 to 10 minutes. Similarly, there should be a "cool-down" period that should also last 5 to 10 minutes and gradually bring the heart rate down to pre-exercise levels.

E. Issues specific to people with diabetes. The use of silica gel or air midsoles as well as polyester or blend (cotton plus polyester) socks to prevent blisters and keep the feet dry is important in minimizing trauma. Patients must be taught to monitor closely for blisters both before and after exercise. During exercise, fluid should be taken early and often.

F. Guidelines for blood glucose management during exercise in type 1 diabetes

1. Avoid exercise if fasting glucose levels are >250 mg/dL and ketosis is present. Caution should be taken if glucose levels are >300 mg/dL and no ketones are present. This is because these levels of hyperglycemia are seen with severe insulin deficiency, and in the environment of exercise with a counterregulatory hormone increase, significant ketosis could ensue.

2. Ingest added carbohydrate if glucose levels are below 100 mg/dL.

3. Determine blood glucose levels before and after exercise.

G. Guidelines for blood glucose management during exercise in type 2 diabetes

1. For patients receiving insulin, **the guidelines are similar, although insulin deficiency is usually not severe** enough to cause ketosis with strenuous exercise.

   2. The dose of insulin secretagogue may need to be decreased, including on the days of exercise.
   3. Oral carbohydrate should always be available in the event of hypoglycemia.

SELECTED READING

American Diabetes Association. Evidence-based nutrition principles and recommendations for the treatment and prevention of diabetes and related complications. *Diabetes Care* 2002;25(suppl 1):S50–S60.

American Diabetes Association. Diabetes mellitus and exercise. *Diabetes Care* 2002;25(suppl 1):S64–S68.

Franz MJ, Bantle JP, Beebe CA, et al. Evidence-based nutrition principles and recommendations for the treatment and prevention of diabetes and related complications. *Diabetes Care* 2002;25:S136–S138.

McNulty SJ, Ur E, Williams G. A randomized trial of sibutramine in the management of obese type 2 diabetic patients treated with metformin. *Diabetes Care* 2003;26:125–131.

Wasserman DH, Zinman B. Exercise in individuals with IDDM. *Diabetes Care* 1994;17:924–937.

Part 1. Pharmacologic Therapy: The Oral Agents

If lifestyle modification is unsuccessful in managing glycemic control in type 2 diabetes to goal, then pharmacologic intervention is indicated. Newly diagnosed type 1 diabetes will obviously require immediate pharmacologic intervention, but the type 2 diabetic patient might only transiently need pharmacologic intervention to treat hyperglycemia associated with metabolic stressors such as surgery or illness, allowing this medication to be discontinued or changed when the patient's own basal β-cell function is no longer stressed. Type 2 diabetes is a combination of metabolic defects—resistant to insulin effect and deficient insulin production. This combination of defects progressively affects insulin secretion; therefore, most patients with type 2 diabetes will eventually require insulin therapy, as endogenous insulin production continues to decrease. As reported in the U.K. Diabetes Prospective Study (UKDPS), typically 50% of β-cell production of insulin has already been lost at the time the diagnosis of diabetes is made. Although initially the glucose abnormality consists of elevated postprandial glucose levels, due largely to decreased muscle cell uptake, secondarily there will then be fasting hyperglycemia due to increased hepatic gluconeogenesis. The insulin level necessary to decrease glucose production in the liver is much lower than the level needed to drive glucose into muscle cells. This results in a dissociation of fasting and postprandial glycemic response, with some patients having very normal or even low fasting glucose levels but markedly elevated postmeal glucose levels. Treatment, therefore, can be targeted to address either pre- or postprandial glycemic regulation, although for most patients, both will need to be targeted. There are three major categories of antiglycemic oral agents: insulin secretagogues [sulfonylureas (SUs) and nonsulfonylureas (non-SUs)], insulin sensitizers [which include the separate categories of biguanide and thiazolidinediones (TZDs)], and α-glucosidase inhibitors (Table 5.1-1).

Table 5.1-1. Oral glycemic control agents

Agent	Initial dose (mg)	Maximum dose (mg)	Alc lowering (max %)	Major side effects
Sulfonylureas				
Glipizide	5	20	1.5	Weight gain, hypoglycemia
Glyburide	5	10	1.5	
Glimepiride	4	8	1.5	
Nonsulfonylureas (glitinides)				
Nateglinide	60 t.i.d.	120 t.i.d.	1.0–1.5	Hypoglycemia
Repaglinide	0.5 t.i.d.	4 t.i.d.	1.0–1.5	
Biguanide				
Metformin	500	2,000	1.5	Diarrhea, nausea, lactic acidosis
a-Glucosidase inhibitors				
Acarbose	25 t.i.d.	100 t.i.d.	1.0	Flatulence, gastrointestinal discomfort
Miglitol	50 t.i.d.	100 t.i.d.	1.0	
Thiazolidenediones				
Rosiglitazone	4	8	1.0	Weight gain, edema
Pioglitazone	30	45	1.0	

  I. Insulin secretagogues include the medications
that are most familiar to most practitioners, as the earliest first-generation SU agent has been available since the
1950s. Chlorpropamide, tolbutamide, acetohexamide, and
tolazamide have been largely replaced by the second-gen-
eration agents glyburide, glipizide, and glimepiride. These
have now been joined by the rapid-acting non-SU agents
repaglinide and nateglinide.
  A. Sulfonylureas facilitate insulin release from the
pancreas at lower glucose levels, through direct effects
on the pancreatic β-cell. Although earlier literature
suggested other potential mechanisms of action, with
the release of insulin from the pancreas being a very
short-term effect, the peripheral effects of SUs are more
likely to be due to decreased glucose toxicity from improved glycemic levels. SUs increase circulating insulin
level, and therefore glucose levels fall.
    1. The average decrease in A1c will be 1% to 1.5%.
    2. Among agents currently available, glimepiride
  binds less avidly in cardiac tissues, which contain
  similar potassium adenosine triphosphate channels
  as in β-cells. This has led to the thought that
  glimepiride might be associated with less ischemic
  preconditioning of the myocardium than other SUs,
  although what this means clinically remains unclear.
  Epidemiologic association between hyperinsulinemia
  and cardiovascular disease has been shown; however,
  in the UKDPS, increased mortality was not seen in
  patients in the SU treatment arm. Another often-
  noted concern is the potential for continued β-cell effect to lead to β-cell exhaustion or a more rapid de-
  pletion of insulin secretion than might be expected.
  This has not been definitively shown as an independent effect from the natural decline in β-cell function
  as an underlying mechanism of the pathophysiology
  of diabetes, independent of treatment modality.
    3. More immediately concerning clinical side ef-
  fects are weight gain, typically from 2 to 5 kg (approximately 5 to 10 lb) in a patient population typically already overweight and struggling with weight
  management, and hypoglycemia. This is a particular
  concern in the elderly, patients with irregular eating
  habits, and patients with renal insufficiency. Although metabolized by the liver, clearance is through
  the kidney, so SUs should be used with caution in
  those with either hepatic or renal impairment. The
  potential of hyponatremia is unique to chlorpropamide, with its inherently long half-life.
    4. Optimal dosing will vary depending on the
  agent chosen, but generally glucose decrease plateaus

at about half the maximal recommended dose. Glipizide should be taken at least 30 minutes before
meals, whereas the timed-release form is not meal
sensitive. SUs are Food and Drug Administration
(FDA) approved for monotherapy and in combination
with other oral glycemic control agents and insulin.

B. **Nonsulfonylureas** work according to the same
mechanism as the SUs but have a much shorter half-
life. These agents have less potential risk of hypoglycemia and therefore less weight gain. Particularly
suited to enhance postprandial insulin release, they are
to be taken before each meal. Multiple daily doses are
required, so convenience is an issue.

    1. A1c maximally lowered by 1% to 1.5%, similar
to action of SUs.

    2. Also need to be used with caution in patients
with hepatic and renal insufficiency as metabolized
by the liver and cleared by the kidney.

    3. Nateglinide does not stimulate insulin secretion
when taken in a fasting state.

    4. FDA approved for monotherapy or with
biguanide.

    5. Are considerably more expensive than SUs.

II. **Insulin sensitizers** include the biguanide metformin and the TZDs pioglitazone and rosiglitazone. Metformin has been available in the United States since the
mid-1990s. The mechanism of action is primarily a hepatic effect with reduced glucose production in the presence of insulin. There is no direct pancreatic effect. Increased glucose disposal has been measured but is
thought to be a secondary effect to decreased glucose toxicity and therefore not a direct drug effect. The TZDs are
incompletely understood with regard to their exact mechanism of action. They activate a cellular nuclear receptor
known as peroxisome proliferator-activated receptor-γ
(PPAR-γ), which in turn alters transcription of a variety of
genes that regulate carbohydrate as well as lipid metabolism. Skeletal muscle cells are stimulated to take up glucose, in turn decreasing hepatic glucose production. This
latter effect is noted only at higher doses of the TZDs.
There is no direct pancreatic effect, although insulin levels may be decreased, even more so than with metformin,
through decreased glucose and free fatty acid level stimu-
lation of β-cell function.

A. Metformin lowers A1c maximally by 1% to 1.5%
when used as monotherapy.

    1. Advantage of metformin over the SUs is de-
creased weight gain or even weight loss. Whether
this is due to the diarrhea that can be seen with the
drug or a true appetite-suppressant effect is not

clear, but weight loss, if seen, is modest, in the range of 5 to 6 lb. Some feel that appetite suppression is due to diminished circulating insulin levels. This decrease may also provide a cardiovascular protective advantage, although there are additional cardiovascular benefits through decreased triglyceride and low-density lipoproteins (LDLs), decreased plasminogen activator factor-1, and decreased vascular endothelial reactivity seen with the use of metformin. In a UKDPS subgroup of overweight individuals randomized to either SU or metformin, the metformin-treated patients had a 39% reduction in cardiac events ($p = 0.01$) and a reduction of all macrovascular endpoints by 30% ($p = 0.02$).

2.   The challenge of metformin is to choose those patients for whom this drug will be safe. The risk of lactic acidosis is approximately 1 per 30,000 patient—years of use. It should be avoided in patients with renal insufficiency defined as serum creatinine level of ≥ 1.5 mg/dL for men and ≥ 1.4 mg/dL for women. As decreased renal function might be more difficult to define in the elderly, in whom decreased muscle mass might mask renal insufficiency, care should be also taken in prescribing metformin to any person over the age of 75 years. Additional contraindications are hepatic dysfunction, including active alcoholism and hepatitis, current congestive heart failure or ongoing treatment for congestive failure, metabolic acidosis, and dehydration. It is recommended that metformin be held in the setting of any acute illness, with alternate therapy provided for glucose control, and held for any surgery as well as in those undergoing radiocontrast studies. Generally, it should be held in anyone being admitted to the hospital due to the potential for any of the previous to be either present at hospitalization or planned during the hospital stay.

3.   More typical concerns are the gastrointestinal side effects of diarrhea, nausea, and abdominal discomfort. Loose bowel movements are even more typical than frank diarrhea. These can be minimized by starting metformin at suppertime with food intake and at lowest dose of 250 or 500 mg and titrating up slowly, in weekly increments of 250 to 500 mg. A typical pattern would be as follows:

- Week 1: 500 mg p.o. with supper
- Week 2: 500 mg p.o. at breakfast and supper
- Week 3: 500 mg p.o. at breakfast
  - 1,000 mg p.o. at supper

- Week 4: 1,000 mg p.o. at breakfast
  - 1,000 mg p.o. at supper

Maximum effective dose is typically 2,000 mg per day. A slow-release form is available for once-daily use, although the side effect profile is essentially the same. Doses up to 2,550 total per day can be used (as 850 mg t.i.d.), but tolerance of side effects typically peaks at 2,000 mg.

   4. Metformin is approved for monotherapy, in combination with SUs, non-SUs, TZDs, and insulin. There are combination medication forms available containing glyburide/metformin and recently approved glipizide/metformin and metformin/rosiglitazone. Need for polypharmaceutical approach reflects the known progressive β-cell function loss with type 2 diabetes, as reported in the UKPDS: 50% failing monotherapy after 3 years and 75% after 9 years of treatment.

B. The TZDs maximally lower A1c by 1%.

   1. Additional benefits associated with the TZDs are decreased microalbumin excretion, decreased triglycerides, decreased blood pressure, and enhanced fibrinolysis. Vascular endothelial function is improved through decreased inflammation and decreased smooth muscle cell production. Effect on LDL-cholesterol is more variable, with rosiglitazone increasing LDL-cholesterol, although this has been postulated to be a rise preferentially in more buoyant, less atherosclerotic cholesterol. Carotid intimal thickness has been shown to decrease on ultrasound in diabetic patients treated with pioglitazone. Similar studies done in patients that were taking troglitazone showed the same decrease in carotid intimal thickness, and troglitazone has been shown to decrease neointimal proliferation after coronary angioplasty.

   2. Adverse effects include weight gain that can be in the range of 10 to 30 lb or more. It is difficult to find current estimates of how frequently this occurs; however, initial investigations clearly underestimated the frequency and amount. Recent reports suggest that this effect might be through an enzyme, glycerol kinase, thought to be activated in adipose tissue by TZDs. Weight gain can be both fluid as well as nonfluid. Patients at risk for congestive heart failure are particularly prone to fluid retention. Given that coronary disease is inherently high in all patients with type 2 diabetes, the TZDs should be generally used with caution. They are contraindicated in patients with hepatic insufficiency. A recent report reviewing TZD and the risk of heart failure showed that, after adjusting for confounding variables, the risk of heart failure in patients with initiated TZD therapy was 4.5% as compared with 2.6% in control subjects (hazard ratio 1.61, $p < 0.001$).

   3.   Effective doses of pioglitazone are 30 mg and more typically 45 mg per day. The full benefit of a dose might not be seen for several weeks up to 3 months, so although titration from 15 to 30 mg can be quickly done, a longer period of time should be taken for further titration to allow for full therapeutic effect. Rosiglitazone initial dose is 8 mg daily. The TZDs are approved for monotherapy and in combination with metformin and SUs. Only pioglitazone is approved currently for combined use with insulin. Hepatic function must be monitored monthly, then every 6 months. The TZDs are expensive and, given their side effect potential, are probably not the first choice for treatment. There has been support for the use of TZDs in very early forms of diabetes treatment, given the *potential* for β-cell preservation; however, the ability to determine diabetes duration at the time of typical diagnosis remains elusive at this time.

III.   α-**Glucosidase inhibitors** available currently include acarbose and miglitol. Unlike the previously discussed classes of medication, these act just within the intestinal wall, to block the breakdown of ingested disaccharides and complex carbohydrates. Postprandial hyperglycemia thereby is targeted, potentially affording a cardiovascular effect through decreased triglyceride and insulin levels.

   A.   Anticipated A1c lowering is 0.5% to 1.0%.

   B.   Side effects related to gastrointestinal discomfort, flatulence, and diarrhea can be considerable and typically lead to discontinuance of the medication—if not by the patient, then at the recommendation of the prescribing practitioner after daily phone calls from the patient reporting symptoms. Starting with the smallest dose possible, half of the 50-mg size, and taking several days before adding the next dose can be helpful, but typically a minimum dose of 50 to 100 mg t.i.d. will be required for therapeutic effect.

   C.   Although approved for monotherapy, these agents are more often used in combination with SUs. Whereas these could potentially be more effective as monotherapy in the treatment of early diabetes, due to associated β-cell preservation in clinical trial, their limited efficacy and side effect profile challenge the practitioner.

SELECTED READING

Delea T, Hagiwara M, Edelsberg J, et al. Exposure to glitazone antidiabetics and risk of heart failure among persons with type 2 diabetes: a retrospective population-based cohort analysis. *J Am Coll Cardiol* 2002;39(suppl A):858a–863a(abst).

Inzucchi SE. Oral hypoglycemic therapy for type 2 diabetes. *JAMA* 2002;287:360–372.

Lebovitz HE. Oral therapies for diabetic hyperglycemia. *Endocrinol Metab Clin North Am* 2001;30:909–933.

Nathan DM. Initial management of glycemia in type 2 diabetes mellitus. *N Engl J Med* 2002;347:1342–1349.

Raptis SA, Dimitris GD. Oral hypoglycemic agents: insulin secretagogues, alpha-glucosidase inhibitors and insulin sensitizers. *Exp Clin Endocrinol Diabetes* 2001;109(suppl 2):265–287.

Part 2. Pharmacologic Therapy: Insulin Therapy

Successful treatment with insulin, for either type 1 or type 2 diabetes, cannot be accomplished without sufficient understanding about how physical activity and diet affect blood glucose levels. Furthermore, it is critical to appreciate that a team of individuals expert in diabetes therapy is required to achieve optimal goals. This team does not need to be located in the same clinic or office as the physician supervising the care, but all team members need to be aware of everyone else's responsibilities. At the least, a diabetes nurse educator and a nutritionist need to be available for routine treatment. Furthermore, these other team members should be *certified diabetes educators*, which guarantees they have the fundamental skills required to teach and manage many aspects of diabetes therapy.

I. Nomenclature
A. Insulin classification. One of the practical problems with insulin treatment in the past is that there has been poor standardization in its nomenclature and implementation (Table 5.2-1). We define three types of insulin: Basal (or background) insulin is that insulin used to suppress hepatic glucose production when food is not eaten. This would include insulin availability overnight during sleep and between meals after food absorption. Prandial (or bolus) insulin is that insulin provided to maintain glycemia associated with meals. This is related to glucose disposal at the muscle. The last type of insulin is correction (also called supplemental) insulin, which is that insulin provided to correct hyperglycemia. Correction insulin may be used before meals, between meals, or even for patients with type 2 diabetes not usually receiving insulin. A correction dose of insulin needs to be differentiated from an adjustment. The former relates to short-acting or rapid-acting insulins and is used to correct the blood glucose usually at the time of the injection. The latter refers to any type of insulin and is defined by a change in dose based on a

Table 5.2-1. Definitions of insulin therapy

Basal insulin replacement (also called background insulin): that insulin used to suppress hepatic glucose production when food is not being absorbed (between meals and overnight)

Prandial insulin replacement (also called bolus or mealtime insulin): that insulin used to dispose of glucose into muscle after food consumption

Correction insulin (also called supplemental insulin): that insulin used to treat premeal or between-meal hyperglycemia

Adjustment insulin: a change in the base dose of either basal or prandial insulin

Nonphysiologic insulin replacement: a program of insulin replacement, usually consisting only of basal insulin, where the insulin administration does not attempt to mimic normal insulin secretion. Examples include bedtime NPH insulin, twice-daily NPH insulin, and bedtime insulin glargine injections

Physiologic insulin replacement: a program of insulin replacement, consisting of both basal and prandial insulin, where the insulin administration attempts to mimic normal insulin secretion. Examples include morning and bedtime NPH insulin with premeal regular insulin or bedtime insulin glargine with premeal insulin lispro

consistent pattern of blood glucose levels. For example, for someone taking bedtime NPH insulin with frequent fasting hypoglycemia, the adjustment would be to decrease the dose of bedtime insulin.

B. Insulin programs. As there are only three types of insulin, there are only two strategies for insulin replacement (Table 5.2-1). We refer to nonphysiologic insulin replacement as those regimens that do not try to mimic normal β-cell secretion, such as one injection of NPH insulin at bedtime. *Physiologic insulin replacement* refers to those regimens that have some resemblance of normal insulin secretion. There are now many choices for this type of insulin strategy. In general, physiologic regimens depend on separate replacement of basal insulin and prandial insulin. Traditionally, NPH was our primary basal insulin, and regular was our primary prandial insulin. However, the basal/prandial definitions do not strictly apply with these two insulin preparations. Because of the pharmacokinetics and pharmacodynamics of both of these insulins, we would use each preparation as both a basal and a prandial insulin.

Table 5.2-2. Currently available insulin preparations

Insulin preparation	Onset of action (h)	Peak action (h)	Effective duration of action (h)	Maximum duration (h)
Rapid-acting analog				
Insulin lispro (Humalog)	¼–½	½–1½	3–4	4–6
Rapid-acting analog				
Insulin aspart (NovoLog)	¼–½	½–1½	3–4	4–6
Short acting				
Regular (soluble)	½–1	2–3	3–6	6–8
Intermediate acting				
NPH (isophane)	2–4	6–10	10–16	14–18
Intermediate acting				
Lente (insulin zinc suspension)	3–4	6–12	12–18	16–20
Long acting				
Ultralente (extended insulin zinc suspension)	6–10	10–16	18–20	20–24
Long-acting analog				
Insulin glargine (Lantus)	3–4	8–16	18–20	20–24
Combinations				
70/30—70% NPH, 30% regular	½–1	Dual	10–16	14–18
50/50—50% NPH, 50% regular	½–1	Dual	10–16	14–18
Combination analogs				
75/25—70% NPL, 25% insulin lispro	¼–½	Dual	10–16	14–18
70/30—70% NPH, 30% insulin aspart	¼–½	Dual	10–16	14–18

NPL, neutral protamine lispro.

C. Challenges with standard insulins. Available insulins are noted in Table 5.2-2. The traditional classification of insulin preparations as rapid acting, short acting, intermediate acting, and long acting does not take into account the fact that regular and NPH insulin often act as both prandial and basal insulin. For example, the classic twice daily "split mix" of NPH and regular insulin could be considered a physiologic insulin regimen. The regular insulin would be responsible for peripheral glucose disposal for the breakfast and dinner meals (Fig. 5.2-1). However, due to the long duration of action of this insulin, it also needs to be considered a prandial insulin at lunch. Furthermore, the morning NPH insulin would be a basal insulin after breakfast and lunch absorption, but because of its relatively quick onset, it also needs to be considered part of the prandial insulin component for breakfast (Fig. 5.2-1). The morning NPH is also the primary prandial insulin for lunch. This regimen therefore uses both insulin preparations for both prandial and basal components and, perhaps more importantly, requires strict consistency as to the timing of the injections and the meals. A delay of lunch will usually result in hypoglycemia, at least for many trying to achieve meticulous glycemic control. In fact, due to the overlapping of the NPH and regular insulin in the later part of the morning, many require midmorning snacks to prevent hypoglycemia. More patients have found that using a prandial insulin for each meal (either regular insulin, insulin lispro, or insulin aspart) and a separate basal insulin (NPH, lente, ultralente, or insulin glargine) adds tremendous flexibility to the reg-

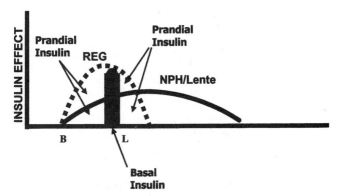

Fig. 5.2-1. **Idealized absorption characteristics of NPH and regular insulin administered prior to breakfast. Note that both insulin types act as both a prandial and a basal insulin.**

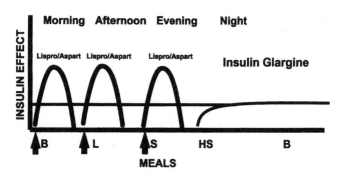

Fig. 5.2-2.   **Modern-day insulin regimen of separate basal and prandial insulins. Insulin glargine is the basal insulin, whereas either insulin lispro or aspart may act as the prandial insulin.**

imen (Fig. 5.2-2). However, for some patients, it is thought to be more inconvenient due to an increased number of injections. Furthermore, except for insulin glargine, for the other basal insulins, it is often difficult to separate how much of an individual injection may have a significant prandial component. General dosing guidelines are noted in Table 5.2-3.

D.   Specific situations: type 1 diabetes (severe insulin deficiency)

1.   With severe insulin deficiency, specific replacement of prandial and basal insulin components is required. As noted above and in Fig. 5.2-1, traditional insulin therapy with twice-daily NPH and regular insulin requires using both insulin components to replace both prandial and basal insulins. In someone with type 1 diabetes and no endogenous insulin secretion, it is difficult, if not impossible, to safely reach target glycemia (HbA1c below 7%) with this regimen. Moving the dinnertime NPH to bedtime was one strategy that attempted to reduce the risk of nocturnal hypoglycemia, but the midday dilemmas related to using the morning NPH and regular as both basal and prandial insulins remained.

2.   Using regular insulin before each meal with NPH at bedtime improves flexibility for mealtimes. Often, a small dose of NPH insulin could be taken in the morning. This regimen gave the most flexibility in the era before insulin analogs.

3.   With the introduction of insulin lispro and later insulin glargine and aspart, it became possible to separate the basal and prandial insulin components. As a general rule of thumb, half the in-

Table 5.2-3. General insulin dosing recommendations

Diabetes type	Basic insulin program	Final dose of insulin (U/kg)	Amount of basal insulin (%)
Type 1	Physiologic replacement	0.4–0.8	50[a]
Type 2	Nonphysiologic regimen	0.3–0.6[b]	100
Type 2	Physiologic regimen	0.3–1.5	50[a]

[a]Assuming basal/bolus regimen with glargine and lispro/aspart or continuous subcutaneous insulin infusion; prandial insulin dose will be based on amount of food at each meal. Nutrition consultation is strongly encouraged, although most type 1 patients will require approximately 1 U of insulin/15 g of carbohydrate, with type 2 patients requiring closer to 1 U/10 g of carbohydrate. The proportion of NPH insulin in those regimens is more variable, based on the amount of NPH used as prandial insulin; yet, the final total dose of insulin will be the same.

[b]Start with 10 U of NPH or insulin glargine at bedtime; increase based on fasting blood glucose.

sulin is used as basal insulin, while the other half is used as prandial insulin (Table 5.2-3). The amount of prandial insulin for each meal can initially be calculated by estimating the approximate amount of calories consumed at each meal. With further nutrition education, it becomes possible to alter the prandial dose by estimating the amount of carbohydrate eaten at each meal or snack. Most of the data evaluating the insulin analogs do so using a standard insulin as the "companion" insulin (e.g., the studies comparing insulin lispro with regular insulin used NPH as the companion as opposed to insulin glargine). It is therefore not surprising that A1c levels in general did not decrease in the original studies. However, as a rule, less hypoglycemia was seen with all of the analog (lispro, aspart, and glargine) studies. This issue becomes much more relevant in people attempting meticulous control (A1c < 7%) or those with hypoglycemia unawareness. Furthermore, the greatest benefit for the newer analogs occurs when both a basal and a prandial analog are used together, although large studies with this combination are not yet available.

   a. The role of snacks. With the use of NPH and regular insulin regimens, snacks are required as part of the program due to the insulin action that occurs between meals. With insulin glargine used as the basal insulin and insulin lispro or aspart as the prandial component, snacks are generally not required. On the other hand, with the use of these analogs, snacks generally require a separate injection of prandial insulin.

4.   Correction insulin. The amount of correction insulin can be determined only by knowing the capillary blood glucose level and the approximate total daily insulin dose (Table 5.2-4).

5.   Insulin pump therapy (continuous subcutaneous insulin infusion). The "gold standard" for physiologic insulin replacement continues to be continuous subcutaneous insulin infusion (CSII). By using only regular insulin or a rapid-acting insulin analog, an external pump delivers basal insulin requirements, usually ranging from 0.5 to 1.5 U per hour. Prandial insulin (traditionally called bolus insulin) is then administered by activating the pump prior to eating. Because the pump is attached with a subcutaneous catheter, between-meal hyperglycemia is much more convenient to correct.

   a. Basic theory. The basic theory of the pump has not changed in the last 25 years: Basal insulin

Table 5.2-4.   Correction dose insulin

Use only regular, aspart, or lispro.

Initial doses

> For regular insulin, "1,500 Rule": 1,500/total daily dose
> = blood glucose in mg/dL; 1 U will decrease blood glucose.
>
> For insulin lispro or aspart, "1,800 Rule": 1,800/total daily
> dose = blood glucose in mg/dL; 1 U will decrease blood glucose.

is provided based on individual requirements, but compared with basal insulin provided by NPH or even insulin glargine, basal insulin infusion with CSII can be programmed to change. This can be advantageous for the morning insulin resistance, which is challenging for some patients (the "dawn phenomenon"), or the decrease in insulin requirements that occurs with exercise. One consistent finding in studies examining CSII has been the decrease in hypoglycemia seen compared with multiple injections.

   b.   Insulin use with continuous subcutaneous insulin infusion. It is clear that either insulin lispro or insulin aspart is superior to regular insulin in a CSII program. The majority of patients tend to require less insulin on CSII than when receiving multiple injections. Most clinicians decrease the dose by 20% to 30% when initiating pump therapy and then use 50% of the final dose as basal insulin. It has been observed that many adolescents may require about 60% of the total dose as prandial insulin.

E.   Specific situations: type 2 diabetes (mild to moderate insulin deficiency). For patients who have exhausted options for oral agents, a nonphysiologic regimen with basal insulin alone may be tried. In general, this works best when the A1c level is below 9%. There is great controversy as to what to do when starting insulin with the oral agents. It is reasonable to maintain the sulfonylurea when no prandial insulin is used. Metformin works extremely well with insulin therapy and in many will prevent additional weight gain. The use of thiazolidinediones with insulin is more problematic as significant weight gain and edema are more common. In fact, only pioglitazone has an indication with insulin use.

   1.   There are several options for basal insulin alone at bedtime. Bedtime insulin glargine has the theoretical advantage of lasting longer to potentially control glycemia long after NPH or ultralente has dissipated. Initial results of a randomized controlled trial showed that with an initial A1c of 8.6%, both bedtime insulin glargine and NPH insulin could, on average, reduce A1c levels to target (6.9%). However, there was less hypoglycemia seen when insulin glargine was used, presumably due to the lack of "peak" with the analog. This study gives a model on how to do this in a practical manner in a busy primary care office. Ten units of insulin are used at bedtime, and the dose is increased every few days until the fasting blood glucose level is normalized.

2.   **When basal insulin alone does not adequately control blood glucose levels, using at least two daily injections will be required.** There are many options for this. Many patients with type 2 diabetes who have not yet progressed to severe insulin deficiency can do well, for a period of time, on twice-daily NPH and regular insulin. Alternatively, many of these patients may be tried on a premixed insulin analog (see Table 5.2-2). It is important to teach patients about using a correction dose of insulin for premeal hyperglycemia, even if they are using a premixed insulin.

F.   **Special situations: type 2 diabetes (severe insulin deficiency).** Patients whose diabetes is not controlled (A1c > 8%) with twice-daily NPH and regular or premixed insulin will need to be treated with similar strategies as patients with type 1 diabetes. The difference between those with type 1 diabetes is the use of the oral agents. At this more advanced stage, there does not appear to be much benefit from the use of the insulin secretagogues. Metformin probably does assist with weight maintenance, and the thiazolidinediones have the problems noted previously with weight gain and edema in this situation. Until long-term studies with these patients are completed, the best use of these oral agents with insulin therapy will be unclear. Many would argue that from an economic point of view, the best advice would be to use generic metformin in combination with insulin or insulin alone for this patient population.

SELECTED READING

Bergenstal RM. Optimization of insulin therapy in patients with type 2 diabetes. *Endocr Pract* 2000;6:93–97.

Bolli GB, DiMarchi RD, Park GD, et al. Insulin analogues and their potential in the management of diabetes mellitus. *Diabetologia* 1999;42:1151–1167.

Buse JB. The use of insulin alone and in combination with oral agents in type 2 diabetes. *Primary Care* 1999;26:931–950.

Herbst KL, Hirsch IB. Insulin strategies for primary care physicians. *Clin Diabetes* 2002;20:11–17.

Hirsch IB. Type 1 diabetes and the use of flexible insulin regimens. *Am Fam Physician* 1999;60:2343–2356.

Owens DR, Zinman B, Bolli GB. Insulins today and beyond. *Lancet* 2001;358:739–746.

Riddle MC. Timely addition of insulin to oral therapy for type 2 diabetes. *Diabetes Care* 2002;25:395–396.

Skyler JS. Insulin therapy in type II diabetes: who needs it, how much of it, and for how long? *Postgrad Med* 1997;101:85–96.

Part 3. Pharmacologic Therapy: Supplements and Alternative Therapies for the Treatment of Diabetes

It has been documented that over one-third of Americans use some form of unconventional therapy, and about one-third of these people saw providers for their therapies. No one has determined how many patients with diabetes use complementary therapies. There was one survey published in 1994 from the United Kingdom showing that patients with diabetes would, on occasion, use herbal treatments instead of conventional medications, and the result included an increase in complications, hospitalizations, ketoacidosis, and acute hyperglycemia. Nevertheless, it is clear that there are many alternative therapies that have benefit for the appropriate patient. As these therapies are so accessible, particularly with the use of the Internet, it is often challenging to stay abreast of therapies our patients may use. By definition, complementary and alternative medicine (CAM) is any therapy that has not been scientifically tested, which is further defined as having "rigorous evidence of safety and efficacy, as required by the Food and Drug Administration (FDA) for the approval of drugs." Therefore, what may be considered CAM can change, as therapies are proven safe and effective with appropriately controlled clinical trials. The National Institutes of Health is now funding millions of dollars of research in CAM, including biological therapies, manipulative and body-based therapies, alternative systems of healing, mind–body medicine, and energy medicine.

I. Select micronutrients in diabetes management
A. Chromium. The trace element chromium is required for the maintenance of normal glucose metabolism. Experimental chromium deficiency leads to impaired glucose tolerance, which improves when chromium is restored to the diet. Usual dietary intake of chromium in the United States is between 20 and 30

µg per day. There is no evidence that people with diabetes have increased rates of deficiency, although the osmotic diuresis that occurs with poorly controlled diabetes makes this population at risk for deficiency for all micronutrients. The current evidence suggests that chromium improves insulin resistance, but the exact mechanism of how this may occur is not clear. The most definitive support for chromium supplementation comes from a 1997 randomized, double-blind, placebo-controlled study conducted in China. Subjects received either placebo or chromium picolinate at either 200 or 1,000 µg per day. After 4 months, there was a clear dose–response for improvements of hemoglobin A1c (A1c) and lipid levels. How applicable this study is to American patients with diabetes is unclear as usual dietary chromium, ethnicity, and body mass index are all different from those in the subjects in the Chinese study. Upon examination of all the data, the results of the studies are mixed. Studies using higher doses and more bioavailable forms of chromium have had more positive effects than those using other forms of chromium. Toxicity of chromium is low, although there are case reports of renal and hepatic toxicity, psychiatric disturbances, and hypoglycemia with large doses of drug. As accurate biochemical indexes of chromium status are not available, assessment of status and responsiveness to supplementation can be established only by trial. Positive effects should be noted within 6 to 12 weeks of supplementation. Most recommend that if clear benefit is not established, the supplement should be discontinued owing to the possibility of as-yet-unidentified toxicities. Most authors do not suggest supplements in excess of >200 µg per day. The American Diabetes Association (ADA) does not recommend chromium supplementation for people with diabetes.

B. Vanadium. The trace element vanadium has not been established as an essential nutrient, and human deficiency has not been documented. Vanadyl sulfate and sodium metavanadate are the most common supplemental forms, but other organic vanadium compounds have been developed. Vanadium acts primarily as an insulin-mimetic agent, although enhanced insulin activity and increased insulin sensitivity have also been noted. Glucose clamp studies in subjects with type 2 diabetes have found increases in insulin sensitivity in some but not all cases. One study showed a decrease in insulin requirement in subjects with type 1 diabetes. Unfortunately, relatively small doses of supplemental vanadium are potentially toxic. Patients using oral supplements most commonly report nausea, vomiting, cramping, flatulence, and diarrhea. These effects are transient and improve with a decrease in dose. Long-term use has been associated with anorexia, decreased food and fluid intake, and weight loss. Vanadium may also enhance the activity of digoxin and anticoagulant medications. Because of these concerns and the lack of information on the long-term effects of pharmacologic doses of vanadium, it is not recommended for use to treat diabetes. Current research is working on forms of vanadium that are better absorbed with fewer side effects.

C.   Nicotinamide/niacin. Nicotinamide/niacin (vitamin B_3) occurs in two forms: nicotinic acid and nicotinamide. Nicotinic acid is used for the treatment of dyslipidemia, although it is has never been a first-line therapy owing to its worsening of insulin resistance. Recently, nicotinamide was reported to be ineffective for the prevention of type 1 diabetes in high-risk individuals in the European Nicotinamide Diabetes Intervention Trial. Studies to date have not found it to be effective at improving diabetes control.

D.   Magnesium. This mineral functions as an essential co-factor for >300 enzymes. Magnesium deficiency has been associated with hypertension, insulin resistance, glucose intolerance, dyslipidemia, cardiovascular disease, diabetes complications, and complications of pregnancy. The causal role of magnesium deficiency in these disorders is not known. Although blood magnesium is commonly measured in the clinical laboratory, <0.3% of the total body magnesium is found in the serum. This makes assessment of true magnesium status difficult as low serum magnesium is a specific, but not a sensitive, indicator of magnesium deficiency. Magnesium deficiency is extremely common in diabetes, especially when poorly controlled due to urinary magnesium losses. Diuretic and alcohol use are the other two most common etiologies of hypomagnesemia, and patients with poorly controlled diabetes who have these other two risk factors are particularly susceptible to low magnesium levels. Clinical trials evaluating the effect of supplemental magnesium on glycemic control and hypertension are mixed. Most trials have shown little effect of magnesium on lipid levels. It is interesting that studies evaluating magnesium status in patients with diabetic retinopathy have found lower magnesium levels, but a cause-and-effect relationship cannot be concluded and there have been no placebo-controlled replacement trials for this group. Furthermore, one could speculate the magnesium is lower in this population because of the greater degree of hyperglycemia and glycosuria, making these patients more susceptible to the retinopathy in the first place. With normal renal function, magnesium is nontoxic. Chronic supplementation in patients with renal insufficiency can lead to magnesium toxicity, resulting in hypotension, headaches, nausea, altered cardiac function, and central nervous system disorders. Currently, the ADA recommends assessment of magnesium status in patients at risk for deficiency and supplementation for documented deficiencies. Oral supplements are available in several forms, but some research suggests that magnesium citrate is more bioavailable. Supplements up to 350 mg per day are appropriate. Often, patients may be started on these higher doses but after a few weeks can be maintained on lower doses. In patients with renal insufficiency, supplementation must be monitored closely.

E.   Vitamin E. This essential fat-soluble vitamin functions primarily as an antioxidant. Antioxidants have been proposed as preventative and treatment agents for many diseases such as cardiovascular disease and cancer. There are some data to suggest that people with diabetes have greater antioxidant requirements because of increased free radical production with hyperglycemia. Unfortunately, despite some positive trials, the largest randomized, controlled trial in people with diabetes receiving vitamin E or placebo showed no benefit of 400 IU of natural vitamin E per day compared with placebo after 4.5 years. There are data to suggest vitamin E improves low-density lipoprotein (LDL) oxidation, but positive effects may be greater for buoyant LDL than for the dense LDL seen in type 2 diabetes. Data showing changes in glycemic control and insulin resistance with vitamin E are mixed. Vitamin E is relatively nontoxic, although it does have some antioxidant properties; thus, patients using medications or supplements known to decrease blood clotting, such as warfarin, aspirin, gingko biloba, garlic, and ginseng, may be at increased risk for bleeding with high-dose supplements. It is thought that doses of 400 IU are safe whereas doses above 800 IU alter blood clotting, although trials to date have not noted changes in prothrombin times. One study has actually noted an increase risk of hemorrhagic stroke (and a decreased risk of ischemic stroke) in smokers. The ADA does not recommend regular supplementation of vitamin E in people with diabetes.

F.   Ginseng. A variety of products are called ginseng. The most common ones used are three different botanicals: Asian, Russian, and American ginseng. The part used is the root. In diabetes, only American and Asian ginseng have been well studied. Ginseng has been studied only in type 2 diabetes. At best, the results have been mixed. For example, one study showed a statistical decrease in fasting blood glucose level with 100 mg per day of ginseng but not 200 mg per day. Other studies have shown no differences. Evidence for efficacy of ginseng is quite limited.

G.   Aloe. This is a desert plant with a cactus-like appearance. There are >500 species, but the most common one is aloe vera. It has been used since prehistoric times for burns and wound healing. There are two types of aloe vera: aloe gel and aloe juice. The gel is used topically but has been used orally for diabetes. The hypoglycemic effect of the oral gel is mild at best and may cause abdominal cramps, diarrhea, pain, and severe electrolyte abnormalities. There are no controlled trials reported with aloe, but one uncontrolled study noted an A1c reduction of 10.6% to 8.2%. Until further studies are reported, this agent cannot be recommended as a supplement for people with diabetes.

II.   Products that may treat the complications of diabetes

A.   γ-Linolenic acid. γ-Linolenic acid (GLA) is an ω-6 fatty acid. The main source for this is evening primrose oil. GLA has been used to treat diabetic neuropathy in addition to a host of other conditions. There have been two trials using GLA. One was a randomized, double-blind study that included subjects with both type 1 and type 2 diabetes. In this trial, at the end of 6 months, there was an improvement in neuropathy symptom scores for the group receiving 360 mg per day of GLA. There was also an improvement in neuropathy symptom scores in the second study for those patients with initial A1c levels below 10%. A1c levels did not change with the GLA in either study. Although these two studies are interesting and the drug is benign, its role in treating neuropathic complications requires more study.

B.   Ginkgo biloba. This is one of the world's oldest living tree species dating back >200 million years. Active ingredients include flavonoids and terpenoids, consisting of ginkgolides and bilobalides. Clinical studies using these compounds have found improvements in claudication. One meta-analysis found a significant effect on increased pain-free walking distance. There are also some data to suggest ginkgo may improve antidepressant-induced sexual dysfunction. It is usually administered from 120 to 160 mg per day in divided doses. Clearly, more definitive studies are required.

C. Garlic. There are some data to suggest garlic for use in diabetes. One report showed garlic to result in increased serum insulin levels and improved liver glycogen storage. Its main use is for the treatment of hypertension and dyslipidemia. A meta-analysis reported that garlic resulted in a small but significant reduction of serum cholesterol of 16 mg/dL. Similarly small differences have been shown with hypertension. One meta-analysis showed a decrease of systolic blood pressure of 8 mm Hg compared with placebo, whereas diastolic blood pressure was reduced by 5 mm Hg. Doses used are 600 to 900 mg per day in divided doses. Although garlic may have beneficial effects for both cholesterol and blood pressure, it is unlikely this agent will be able to treat these two risk factors to target in people with diabetes who require aggressive therapy. Furthermore, there are no outcome studies with garlic.

D. Folic acid. It is now well accepted that hyperhomocystinemia is correlated with coronary artery disease, stroke, and peripheral vascular disease. Furthermore, it was shown that hyperhomocystinemia is a risk factor for overall mortality in type 2 diabetes. Normal levels of pyridoxine (vitamin B_6), cobalamin (vitamin B_{12}), and folate are required for normal homocysteine metabolism. Folate refers to a family of naturally occurring compounds. Folic acid is the synthetic form of the vitamin. The recommended daily allowance for folate is 400 μg per day for adults and 600 μg per day in pregnancy. Metformin may decrease folate and vitamin B_{12} absorption and increase homocysteine levels. The clinical significance of this effect is not clear. Vitamin B_{12} has been used for years as a treatment of painful neuropathy in diabetes, but there are few data to support this practice. In patients with diabetes and hyperhomocystinemia, increased folate intake decreases and occasionally normalizes homocysteine levels. Unfortunately, there are no definitive data to date showing if supplementation is effective in prevention or treatment of microvascular or macrovascular complications of diabetes. Long-term trials of folate supplementation in patients with diabetes would be welcomed. However, the supplement is extremely safe as doses of <15 mg per day have not been associated with any adverse effects. The main concern with folate supplementation is that it could mask the anemia associated with B_{12} deficiency, resulting in permanent nerve damage. High-dose folate could also interfere with anticonvulsants. High doses of pyridoxine may result in neuropathic pain; thus, this is not suggested for the treatment of diabetic neuropathy. At this time, the only population recommended to take folic acid supplements comprises women of childbearing age, due to the data showing prevention of birth defects. However, all patients with diabetes are encouraged to consume adequate quantities of dietary folate, B_{12}, and B_6 and to modify factors that increase homocysteine levels, such as alcohol intake and smoking. All enriched cereal grain products have been fortified with folic acid in the United States since 1998. Good dietary products for B_{12} include most animal products; B_6 can be found in whole grains, animal products, and legumes.

III.   Summary. The supplements listed in this chapter by no means form a complete list; rather, some of the more common alternative therapies used by people with diabetes were discussed. Less than 40% of patients tell their health care providers they take complementary therapies. Although there are likely many reasons for this, it is important for clinicians to know what products their patients are taking. Interactions with alternative therapies and conventional medications are common; thus, clinicians will need to frequently research unfamiliar therapies. There are currently many questions about how different CAM therapies affect diabetes and its complications. The efficacy and possible adverse events of these therapies will become more evident as randomized, controlled trials are performed.

SELECTED READING

Astin JA. Why patients use alternative medicine: results from a national study. *JAMA* 1998;279:1548–1553.

Gill GV, Redmond S, Garratt F, et al. Diabetes and alternative medicine: cause for concern. *Diabetes Med* 1994;11:210–213.

National Center for Complementary and Alternative Medicine, sponsored by the National Institutes of Health (NIH). Up-to-date information about CAM and clinical trials. *www.nccam.nih.gov.*

Sabo CE, Rush MS, Temple LL. The use of alternative therapies by diabetes educators. *Diabetes Ed* 1999;25:945–956.

Sarubin A. *The health professional's guide to popular dietary supplements.* Chicago: American Diabetes Association, 2000.

Yusuf S, Dagenais G, Pogue J, et al. Vitamin E supplementation and cardiovascular events in high risk patients. The Heart Outcomes Prevention Evaluation Study. *N Engl J Med* 2000; 342:154–160.

Acute Complications of Diabetes Mellitus

Hyperglycemic crises in diabetes mellitus can be thought of as the end result of progressive metabolic decompensation. The classic forms of hyperglycemic crises, diabetic ketoacidosis (DKA) and hyperglycemic hyperosmolar syndrome (HHS), can be clinically more overlapping than two distinctly separate entities. In 200 of 612 patients with decompensated diabetes, features of both DKA and HHS were present. In the same patient, episodes of DKA occurred at times, HHS at other times. For both conditions, treatment goals include correction of the metabolic as well as volume status of the patient, identification of any precipitating and co-morbid conditions, transition to a long-term treatment, and a specific plan to prevent recurrence.

I. **Hyperglycemic hyperosmolar syndrome** is the prototype of hyperglycemic crises in type 2 diabetes mellitus. Estimates of incidence are 1 of every 1,000 hospital admissions and a frequency of 1 in 17.5 cases per 100,000 person–years. Precise mortality data are not available due to the high prevalence of co-morbid disease that is then listed as the main cause of death rather than HHS. Estimates of death range from approximately 60% to as low as 15%, the latter being suggested as due to earlier recognition of illness and treatment initiation because the majority of deaths due to HHS occur within the first 1 to 2 days. Typical clinical presentation is a patient over the age of 50, about one-third with previously undiagnosed diabetes, and a person dependent on others for daily care. About 30% are actually direct admissions from a nursing home, where the presence of multiple co-morbid illnesses, increasing lack of ability of self-care, and predisposition toward dehydration are significant predisposing features for HHS.

A. **Hyperglycemic hyperosmolar syndrome can lead to central nervous system irritability,** which can present as seizure, hemiparesis, confusion, or coma. Coma is much less common than previously thought, whereas lethargy and decreased sensorium are more frequently seen; therefore, HHS can be the etiology of symptoms initially evaluated in an outpatient office setting. Physical exam will usually reveal tachypnea and low-grade fever, with normal blood pressure and respiratory rate. If hypotension is present with fever and tachypnea, infection should be suspected, particularly a gram-negative sepsis. Dehydration manifesting as poor skin tissue turgor may be difficult to appreciate in an elderly individual but can be more commonly appreciated through exam for dryness of buccal mucous membranes. Abdominal distention with nausea, emesis, and pain can be associated with gastroparesis that is not due to autonomic neuropathy but rather hypertonicity. This typically will resolve spontaneously with fluid treatment. Lethargy and disorientation are common. Focal neurologic signs are common in HHS, thought to reflect further cerebrovascular insufficiency in areas of previous flow insufficiency, and can lead to a diagnosis of suspected acute cerebrovascular accident, but findings remit with fluid treatment. Seizures can be seen in up to 25% of patients and can be either focal or generalized. An unusual type of seizure, epilepsia partialis continua, has been reported in up to 6% of HHS patients in the early phase of HHS when a lower osmolality of typically <330 mOsm/L is present. HHS-associated seizures are usually resistant to usual anticonvulsant therapy, and phenytoin commonly used to treat seizures may further exacerbate HHS.

B. Laboratory findings include plasma glucose level of ≥600 mg/dL and serum osmolality of >320 mOsm/kg. Mild acidemia is often present, characterized as arterial pH of >7.30 and serum HCO_3^- level of ≥15 mEq/L. The average serum creatinine and blood urea nitrogen levels are 3.0 and 65 mg/dL, respectively. The osmolality is often roughly calculated as "effective serum osmolality" from corrected (for glucose) sodium, potassium, and glucose, as urea is thought to be equally distributed in body components (Table 6-1). About 50% of patients with HHS will have a mild anion gap metabolic acidosis. When the acidosis is severe, the differential diagnosis should be extended to consider lactic acidosis or other non-HHS entities. Vomiting or use of thiazide diuretic can cause a metabolic *alkalosis* that can mask the severity of the acidosis. This might be suspected when the combined anion gap and measured bicarbonate combining power (HCO_3^-) is higher than normal.

C. Precipitating factors of hyperglycemic hyperosmolar syndrome can be divided into several

Table 6-1. Useful formulas for the evaluation and treatment of hyperglycemic hyperosmolar syndrome

Calculation of the effective serum osmolality

Effective P_{OSM} = 2 × ([Na$^+$] + [K$^+$]) + [glucose (mg/dL)/18]

Corrected serum sodium

Corrected [Na$^+$] = [Na$^+$] + 1.6 × ([glucose (mg/dL)] − 100)/100

---

groupings (Table 6-2) including infectious, co-existing illness, and medication.

   1. Infections are most frequent, with estimates ranging from 32% to as high as 60%, with pneumonia, urinary tract infection, and sepsis seen most often. This has led to recommendations to start antibiotic therapy early in HHS treatment protocols, even if an infectious agent or source has not been identified; others recommend waiting for more definite evidence, as both fever and leukocytosis can be frequently seen in all episodes of HHS. Concurrent medical illnesses can include vascular occlusive illness such as silent myocardial infarction, cerebrovascular disease, pulmonary embolus, and mesenteric thrombosis.

   2. Metabolic illnesses implicated as precipitating factors for HHS include acute pancreatitis, intestinal obstruction, renal failure (also peritoneal dialysis either by the contraction of effective arterial blood volume or by development of secondary pancreatitis), severe burns, hypothermia, and heat stroke. Endocrine causes include thyrotoxicosis, Cushing's syndrome, acromegaly, as well as previously undiagnosed diabetes mellitus. Even ectopic production of adrenocorticotrophic hormone from tumor has been reported.

   3. Medications recently have become increasingly the precipitating agents of HHS, particularly ones not uncommonly prescribed for the older population and ones known to inhibit the secretion or action of insulin. These include thiazide as well as loop diuretics, calcium-channel blockers, diazoxide, and propranolol. Glucocorticoids, immunosuppressive drugs, and L-asparagine have been reported, as well as phenytoin and chlorpromazine. Cimetidine has been associated with HHS. Total parenteral nutrition has been reported as a precipitating factor for HHS, although these patients tended to have either a very positive family history of diagnosed diabetes or themselves a past medical history of diabetes mellitus.

Table 6-2. Categories of conditions associated with hyperglycemic hyperosmolar syndrome and diabetic ketoacidosis

Infection	Co-existing illness	Medications	Endocrine	Other
Pneumonia	Renal failure	Diuretics: thiazide, loop	Thyrotoxicosis	Heat stroke
Urinary tract infection	Intestinal obstruction	β-Blockers	Glucocorticoid excess	Severe burns
	Acute pancreatitis	Calcium channel blockers		Hypothermia
Sepsis	Myocardial infarction	Cimetidine	Acromegaly	Postop: ortho, cardiac
		Glucocorticoids	Undiagnosed diabetes mellitus	Chemical abuse: alcohol, cocaine
		Phenytoin		
		Antipsychotics		
		Total parenteral nutrition		
		Missing insulin, oral agent doses		

Noncompliance with intake of diabetes medication has been reported as a contributing cause in up to 25% of patients with HHS. Postoperative patients also have a high risk of HHS, particularly those having undergone orthopedic and cardiac bypass surgery, thought to be due to procedure-associated increases in intravenous osmotic load with dextrose-containing fluids. Neurosurgical procedures have been associated with development of HHS, although whether this is due to direct central nervous system injury, solute load, or the concurrent use of medications that independently have been associated with HHS, such as glucocorticoids or phenytoin, remains unclear. Similar issues have been raised in the understanding of HHS developing with various other surgical procedures such as renal transplantation.

D.   Treatment of hyperglycemic hyperosmolar syndrome is targeted at fluid replacement, and this is best done in an inpatient setting. Rapid volume repletion is required both for patient survival as well as to decrease the high risk of thromboembolism. The magnitude of fluid required will vary from individual to individual, but deficits of about 20% to 25% body water, about 12% body weight, or about 9 L are typical in HHS. Initial fluid replacement should consist of 1 to 2 L over the first 2 hours of treatment, followed by 7 to 9 L over the next 2 to 3 days, with specific rate and type of fluid determined individually. There remains controversy over the ideal fluid replacement choice: isotonic or hypotonic. Normal saline has the advantage of more quickly replacing intracellular volume, yet thereby increasing the risk of fluid overload in patients with potential cardiac and respiratory compromise and consequent complication of adult respiratory distress syndrome. Hypotonic fluids such as 0.45% saline can be more effective at replacing free water loss but thereby increase the risk of too rapid correction of hypernatremia with the potential for diffuse myelinolysis and death. A compromise seems to be starting fluid replacement with normal saline, up to 1 L, then switching to 0.45% saline when urine output is well established, with the goal of replacing half of the free water deficit in the initial 12 hours of therapy and the remaining half over the next 12 hours. Once serum glucose drops below 250 mg/dL, it is recommended that glucose be added to the intravenous fluids. The rare reports of cerebral edema in HHS have all occurred when serum glucose fell below 250 mg/dL.

   1.   Colloids are not recommended as replacement fluids, as they can contribute to an already high

plasma viscosity and exacerbate vascular insufficiency, unless shock occurs despite maximal replacement with isotonic fluids.

2.   In the established end-stage renal failure patient, fluid replacement has little role, and treatment
modalities are limited to correction of electrolyte abnormalities and providing insulin.

3.   Once fluid replacement is initiated, attention
then should be turned to electrolyte balance. There is
a significant expectant diuresis of sodium, potassium,
magnesium, calcium, and phosphate in HHS.

   a.   Replacement of potassium takes precedence,
   although hyperkalemia is often present initially.
   Normokalemia or hypokalemia suggests a potassium deficit between minimally 3 and as much as
   10 mEq/kg. Severe hypokalemia is more often associated with history of use of thiazide diuretic, naso-
   gastric suction, or emesis. Replacement of potassium should not be started until urine output has
   been established. Initial replacement should consist of between 20 and 40 mEq/L of infused fluid,
   with the goal of maintaining a potassium level of
   3.0 to 5.0 mEq/L. Electrocardiographic monitoring
   is recommended. Potassium can be replaced as
   potassium chloride; there has been no reported clinical advantage in choosing potassium phosphate or
   potassium acetate other than expense.

   b.   Although phosphate, magnesium, and calcium losses do occur in HHS, there are no data
   unique to HHS showing that the replacement of
   these is routinely necessary.

4.   Insulin therapy is clearly a secondary adjunct
to fluid replacement. Recommended doses are similar
to those in DKA, with an initial insulin bolus of 0.1
U/kg followed by intravenous infusion of 0.1 to 0.15
U/kg per hour. Starting insulin therapy before fluid
therapy can shift 2 to 3 L of fluid from intracellular to
extracellular compartments and potentiate hypo-
volemia, shock, and thromboembolism. Fluids alone
can be therapeutic in HHS and can decrease serum
glucose by 80 to 200 mg/dL per hour.

**5.   There is controversy about the routine ini-
tiation of antibiotics, as discussed, and about
the routine initiation of anticoagulant therapy**
in this population at risk for thromboembolic event.
Whereas low-dose heparin has been recommended by
some, the disadvantage of starting prophylactic heparin treatment is potentiating gastrointestinal hemorrhage in the setting of hypertonicity-induced gastroparesis. As a compromise, it has been suggested

that waiting 1 to 2 days before starting heparin would allow gastroparesis to resolve, while then starting heparin only if the patient is expected to remain nonambulatory.

6. Monitoring treatment progress is imperative to successful treatment outcome. Flow sheets, either paper or electronic, are necessary to follow treatment. Coupled with clinical re-evaluation of the patient, this can allow for many patients with HHS not to require the invasive intervention of Swan–Ganz line placement or intra-arterial catheter, which could potentiate infection. Even bladder catheterization should be avoided, if at all possible.

7. As important as the treatment of the acute hyperglycemic crisis is the **planning for interventions to prevent the recurrence of hyperglycemic hyperosmolar syndrome.** Monitoring hydration status, establishing a routine for home glucose monitoring, and providing education for "sick day" treatments have been recommended as preventive measures in the recurrence of HHS.

II. Diabetic ketoacidosis. The annual incidence of DKA in the United States is approximated at 5 to 8 episodes per 1,000 people with diabetes. DKA can be seen in both type 1 and 2 and can be the presenting condition in both types of diabetes. Two percent to 8% of all hospital admissions for diabetes are related to DKA, but with availability of self-blood glucose monitoring, increasingly DKA can be recognized in the early stages and often amenable to treatment in an office or urgent clinic setting. However, mortality rates for DKA have shown little decline from a 2% to 10% range over the last three decades. Mortality rate in the patient over 65 years in particular is significant at excess of 20%, whereas in the younger patient, it is 2% to 4%.

A. In contrast to hyperglycemic hyperosmolar syndrome, DKA in type 2 diabetes is associated with glucose levels typically in the 250- to 500-mg/dL range, a serum osmolality of 300 mOsm/L, and a pH of ≤7.30 with ketonemia. In defining predisposing or associated conditions for the development of DKA for patients with type 2 diabetes, suggested associations include higher body mass index, male gender, history of poorer glycemic control, consistent high carbohydrate intake, and African American, Pacific Asian, and American Indian ethnicity.

Among all patients with DKA, a presenting glucose level of ≤350 mg/dL will be seen in 15%. An increased anion gap ($[Na^+] - [HCO_3^-] - [Cl^-]$) over 10 mEq/L is common. The use of the anion gap with serum bicarbonate and arterial pH has been proposed as a means of categorizing DKA into mild, moderate, and severe categories, with mild DKA constituting an anion gap of >10 mEq/L, serum bicarbonate level of 15 to 18 mEq/L, and arterial pH of 7.25 to 7.30. Severe DKA is considered an anion gap of >12 mEq/L, serum bicarbonate level of <10 mEq/L, and arterial pH of <7.00. However, clinical evaluation of sensorium with particular emphasis on degree of mental obtundation must accompany any laboratory work. Plasma osmolality is typically increased but often does not exceed 320 mOsm/kg. Serum ketones are present at >1:2 dilution. New-onset diabetes is the classic etiology of DKA in type 1 diabetes, but in previously diagnosed diabetes, infection and omission of insulin are the most frequent precipitating factors.

1. **Creatinine levels may be falsely elevated,** as ketone bodies interfere with automated creatinine measurements, particularly acetoacetate.

2. **Serum ketones can be measured qualitatively,** except when lactic acidosis or alcohol excess is suspected, as β-hydroxybutyrate is preferentially the ketone body formed in these patients. Qualitative assays detect acetoacetate and less so acetone but not β-hydroxybutyrate, so ketonemia may be underestimated in these patients.

B.   Clinical presentation includes nausea, polydipsia, polyuria, weakness, and fatigue. Abdominal pain can be seen with exam showing evidence of ileus. This can lead to confusion over a metabolic versus precipitating abdominal etiology of the pain. Current recommendations are first to treat dehydration and metabolic acidosis, then re-evaluate if symptoms and findings persist. Up to 25% of patients with DKA will have emesis, which may resemble coffee grounds and be guaiac positive. Endoscopy has shown this to be due to hemorrhagic gastritis. Kussmaul respirations, hypotension, and tachycardia can be seen. Hypothermia is felt to be a poor prognostic sign.

1. **Differential diagnosis of ketoacidosis** includes starvation ketosis, alcoholic ketoacidosis (which can be distinguished through clinical history), glucose level typically <250 mg/dL, and the presence of hypoglycemia, with serum bicarbonate in alcoholic ketoacidosis rarely <18 mEq/L. Increased anion gap metabolic acidosis besides lactic acidosis can be seen in the ingestion of agents such as salicylates, methanol, ethylene glycol, and paraldehyde. Blood levels of lactate, salicylate, and methanol can help to differentiate these conditions. Urine calcium oxalate and hippurate crystals can be sought in ethylene glycol ingestion. Par-

aldehyde ingestion can be appreciated clinically through its pungent odor on the breath.

C.   Treatment of diabetic ketoacidosis is focused on hydration, insulin use, electrolyte imbalance, and prevention of future episodes. Precipitating causes should be identified and treated concurrently.

1.   Fluid therapy is directed to intravascular and extravascular volume repletion. Isotonic saline of 1 to 2 L in an adult without cardiac compromise over the first hour should then be followed by re-evaluation of fluid status. Subsequent fluid choice, specifically when converted to half-normal saline, will be determined by blood pressure stability, presence of normal or elevated corrected sodium, and clinical exam. Typical body fluid deficit in DKA is 6 L, but overaggressive replacement is associated with the risk of cerebral edema, so after the initial fluid load to clinically stabilize, the fluid rate should be decreased from 15 to 20 to 4 to 14 mL/kg per hour.

a.   In patients younger than 20 years, initial fluid re-expansion should not exceed 50 ml/kg over 4 hours due to increased risk of cerebral edema. A decrease in osmolality of 3 mOsm/kg per hour can be targeted by following the initial 10 to 20 mL/kg per hour the first hour with 5 mL/kg per hour over the next 48 hours, again changing from normal to 0.45% NaCl after the first hour.

b.   Once renal function has been ensured, potassium should be added to fluids, as two-thirds potassium chloride and one-third potassium phosphate.

2.   Insulin constant infusion at a rate of 0.1 U/kg per hour should be started in both pediatric as well as adult patients. Adults should receive an intravenous bolus of 0.15 U/kg after the potassium level has been documented above 3.3 mEq/L. A targeted decrease of 50 to 75 mg/dL per hour is the goal; if this does not occur, insulin infusion can be doubled if hydration status is acceptable. With mild DKA, typically subcutaneous or intramuscular regular insulin given hourly has been shown to be as effective as intravenous infusion, when a priming dose of 0.4 to 0.6 U/kg per hour is first given half subcutaneously, half intramuscularly. Follow-up doses should be decreased to 0.1 U/kg per hour and can be given all in one site.

a.   At a plasma glucose level of 250 mg/dL, the insulin infusion should be decreased to 0.05 to 0.1 U/kg per hour and dextrose added to intravenous fluids, until oral caloric intake is seen and conversion to subcutaneous insulin can be started. Conversion to subcutaneous insulin should be done with some overlap with intravenous infusion. If the patient is taking nothing by mouth, then once the glucose level is ≤200 mg/dL, the serum bicarbonate level is ≥18 mEq/L, and the venous pH is >7.3 (criteria for resolution of DKA), 5 U of regular insulin for every 50 mg/dL over 150 mg/dL, maximally 20 U regular, can be given every 4 hours. If the patient is eating, then an insulin regimen combining basal and prandial insulin should be started, targeting a dose of 0.5 to 1.0 U/kg per day if the patient was not previously on insulin or resuming the previous insulin regimen if indicated.

b. As patients with DKA include those with type 2 diabetes, these patients can possibly be discharged on oral antiglycemic agents. Previously undiagnosed type 2 diabetic patients presenting in DKA need particular monitoring after DKA, as their insulin requirements may drop precipitously following hospitalization. These patients often are unrecognized as having type 2 diabetes until significant hypoglycemia occurs.

3. Treatment complications include cerebral edema, hypoxia, and noncardiogenic pulmonary edema. Cerebral edema occurs in 0.7% to 1.0% of children with DKA. Neurologic deterioration can be rapid, with headache, lethargy, and progressive decrease in arousal, leading to seizures, bradycardia, and respiratory arrest. Once symptoms progress beyond lethargy, a mortality risk of >70% has been reported, and permanent morbidity is seen in 86% to 93%. Reduction in colloid osmotic pressure leading to increased pulmonary water content and decreased lung compliance is associated with hypoxemia. Patients with rales on exam are at higher risk for developing pulmonary edema.

4. Prevention of future DKA episodes, as with HHS, is a critical part of the treatment. Sick day management should be reviewed, with discussion of blood glucose goals as well as when to use specific supplemental insulin doses of short-acting insulin in illness. This should be coupled with review of the need for increased fluid intake, initiation of carbohydrate- and appropriate sodium-containing liquid diet, and when to call the office for help. Education regarding the need to continue insulin, even if caloric intake is diminished, and to check ketones in sustained hyperglycemia and the periodic review of these principles with patients can impact not only individual patient morbidity and survival but also health costs. Repeated admissions for

DKA are estimated to cost 1 of every 2 health care dollars spent on adults with type 1 diabetes.

III.   Diabetes mellitus is associated with many endocrinopathies, which have been associated with exacerbation of hyperglycemia in the established diabetic patient and potentiation of hyperglycemia in those not previously diagnosed. These include acromegaly, hyperprolactinemia, hyperthyroidism, hyperparathyroidism, pheochromocytoma, hyperaldosteronism, and Cushing's syndrome.

A.   Overt diabetes is estimated to occur in 10% to 32% of acromegalic patients, with insulin-like growth factor-1 being a better correlating predictor of the development of diabetes than growth hormone. Successful treatment of acromegaly is associated with variable effect on glucose control, some studies reporting about half of patients having resolution of their diabetes and others either some or no improvement in glycemic control.

B.   Hyperprolactinemia can be associated with mild glucose intolerance, although of questionable clinical significance. Interestingly, treatment of prolactin with bromocriptine has been shown to decrease hyperinsulinemia and improve glucose intolerance and raises a question as to the role of prolactin in the late stages of gestational glucose metabolism.

C.   Hyperthyroidism and diabetes are frequently seen together. Diabetes is twice as prevalent in the hyperthyroid population as in the euthyroid. Treatment of hyperthyroidism typically leads to improved glycemic control, if not frank resolution of glucose intolerance or diabetes.

D.   Pheochromocytoma is associated with a 30% incidence of glucose intolerance. Overt diabetes and ketoacidosis have been reported but are rare, although elevated fasting glucose can be seen in half of the patients. Combined α- and β-adrenergic blockade treatment improves both insulin secretion and glucose tolerance, although only surgical resection of the tumor will result in glucose normalization. This, however, can take weeks to months, due to residual insulin resistance effect.

E.   Ten percent to 29% of patients with **Cushing's syndrome** develop overt diabetes mellitus. Predictors of the development of diabetes in glucocorticoid excess states are age, weight, a family history of diabetes, and a personal history of gestational diabetes, and there is evidence that the more likely person to develop diabetes is the one with decreased insulin secretory reserve. HHS has been reported in patients with Cushing's syndrome and diabetes. Treatment of the hypercortisolism will result often in resolution of diabetes, but not always a return to a euglycemic state.

F. Hyperparathyroidism, when treated in the diabetic individual with surgical removal of affected gland(s), has been associated with improved insulin sensitivity.

G. Glucagonoma patients have an increase in gluconeogenesis but also suppression of insulin secretion contributing to hyperglycemia. When successful surgical resection is possible, the diabetes resolves. Interestingly, although glucagon has been associated with ketosis potential in insulin-deficient states, glucagonoma patients rarely become ketotic.

IV. Medications resulting in hyperglycemia, beyond those mentioned earlier, include the protease inhibitors used to treat patients with human immunodeficiency virus (HIV).

A. In 1% to 6% of HIV-1 patients treated with protease inhibitors, the level of acute hyperglycemia is consistent with that in new-onset type 2 diabetes, whereas many more will show milder impaired glucose tolerance and insulin resistance. The majority does not have diagnosed diabetes prior to the initiation of therapy drug cocktails including protease inhibitor, nor is there a higher incidence of a positive family history of diabetes in these individuals. Hyperglycemia leading to DKA or HHS is not uncommon, and controlling glucose can require insulin therapy. Recent data have suggested that insulin resistance may also be associated with HIV infection, independent of protease treatment, although with discontinuance of protease therapy, there is typically marked metabolic improvement, often with clinical resolution of diabetes. Recombinant growth hormone treatment of muscle wasting in HIV has also been associated with acute hyperglycemia evolving into type 2 diabetes. Pentamidine used in the prevention and treatment of *Pneumocystis carinii* infection has also been associated with hyperglycemia, because of its similarity in appearance to streptozotocin and alloxan, which result in β-cell destruction. The use of this medication results first in hypoglycemia, then hyperglycemia as progressive insulin production and secretion capacity are lost.

B. Niacin can significantly exacerbate hyperglycemia in previously diagnosed diabetes. However, recent literature suggests that this may not be as frequently seen as previously thought, looking at a subpopulation of individuals with diabetes using up to 3 g daily of crystalline niacin for maximum duration of 60 weeks in a dyslipidemia treatment study. In this study, glucose levels increased transiently at the time of niacin initiation and with each dosage increase but subsequently returned to normal. Hemoglobin A1c (A1c) levels did increase slightly, but the change was not statistically significant. Long-acting niacin may cause less hyperglycemia, although data obtained on long-acting forms have been limited to short duration of use.

   C. Antihypertensive medications are commonly used in patients with type 2 diabetes, yet there are numerous reports on the potential diabetogenic effect of diuretics and β-blockers. In individuals with type 2 diabetes, glucose tolerance and fasting glucose deteriorate with initiation of thiazide treatment. In patients with type 1 diabetes, A1c levels can increase with use of doses in the 25- to 50-mg range. This hyperglycemia potentiation effect is not limited to thiazides but has also been reported with the loop diuretic class. Although earlier studies used doses up to 200 mg per day, with subsequent inference that the hyperglycemic effect might be dose mediated, even low doses of thiazide, such as 12.5 to 25 mg/day, have been shown to cause deterioration in glucose tolerance in diabetic individuals. Both decreased insulin sensitivity as well as decreased insulin secretion, the latter possibly mediated through hypokalemia, are postulated mechanisms for the hyperglycemia. For some individuals, however, the ability for compensatory *increased* insulin secretion might offset the insulin resistance.

   1. β-Adrenergic blockers have also been associated with induced hyperglycemia. In patients with type 2 diabetes, reports have shown increased fasting glucose levels as well as increases in A1c levels with β-blocker use. The less specific β-blockers might be more likely to be associated with glucose level deterioration.

   2. Combination of diuretic and β-blocker can result in an even more profound effect on glucose sensitivity and glucose tolerance than either agent alone. In nondiabetic hypertensive subjects, a 10-fold increase of diabetes incidence has been shown in those with this medication combination. In diabetic individuals, both fasting glucose and A1c levels have been shown to increase.

 V. Severe hypoglycemia is defined as an episode requiring the assistance of another person for treatment. It is estimated that after 40 years of type 1 diabetes, an average of 2,000 to 4,000 episodes of symptomatic hypoglycemic episodes can be experienced. Five percent of type 1 diabetic patients die as a result of hypoglycemia, mostly from motor vehicle accidents. According to the Diabetes Control and Complications Trial, 55% of all severe hypoglycemia occurs in sleep. Additional information has suggested a 29% incidence of asymptomatic hypoglycemia (glucose < 53 mg/dL) each night.

A. Contributing factors to hypoglycemia are nonphysiologic insulin delivery, particularly NPH at dinner rather than bedtime, long length of time without food, increased insulin sensitivity at night (not well understood), and position (autonomic symptoms are greater when standing than when supine because of exaggerated epinephrine response in the setting of hypoglycemia and standing). Bedtime calorie ingestion, glucose monitoring between 2:00 and 4:00 A.M., adjustment of timing of intermediate-acting insulin, or even a switch to long-acting basal peakless analog insulin can be helpful in preventing hypoglycemia. Glucose sensor monitoring has been particularly helpful in identifying unrecognized hypoglycemia. Instruction in the use of glucagon both for the patient and for the identified caregiver is effective in treating hypoglycemia, when the patient is asked to designate a caregiver in case of inability to ingest carbohydrate calories.

B. Factors contributing to decisions of in-hospital treatment versus outpatient treatment relate to whether pretreatment was given prior to paramedic evaluation, including either glucagon parenterally or glucose orally, and level of consciousness at the time of paramedic evaluation. In a Danish study, 84% of hypoglycemic patients could be treated at home and remain home, with 6% relapsing within 48 hours and 9% within 72 hours among patients declining transport to hospital.

SELECTED READING

American Diabetes Association Position Statement. Hyperglycemic crises in patients with diabetes mellitus. *Diabetes Care* 2002;(suppl 1):S100–S108.

Anderson PD, Hogskilde J, Wetterslev M, et al. Appropriateness of leaving emergency medical service treated hypoglycemic patients at home: a retrospective study. *Acta Anaesthesiol Scand* 2002;46:464–468.

Bengtsson C, Blohme G, Lapidus L, et al. Do antihypertensive drugs precipitate diabetes? *Br Med J* 1984;289:1495–1497.

Bressler P, DeFronzo RA. Drugs and diabetes. *Diabetes Rev* 1994;1:53–84.

Elam MB, Hunninghake DB, Davis KB. Effect of niacin on lipid and lipoprotein levels and glycemic control in patients with diabetes and peripheral arterial disease. *JAMA* 2000;284:1263–1270.

Genuth S. Hyperosmolar hyperglycemic non-ketotic syndrome (HHNS). In: Lebovitz HE, ed. *Therapy for diabetes mellitus and related disorders,* 3rd ed. Alexandria, VA: American Diabetes Association, 1998:90–96.

Lorber D. Non-ketotic hypertonicity in diabetes mellitus. *Med Clin North Am* 1995;79:39–52.

Trence DL, Hirsch IB. Hyperglycemic crises in diabetes mellitus type 2. *Endocrinol Metab Clin North Am* 2001;30:817–831.

Microvascular and Neuropathic Complications

I. Mechanism of microvascular complications. Possible multifactorial but chronic hyperglycemia is required. Dysregulation of hemodynamic, hormonal, and biochemical factors appears to be involved.

  A. Advanced glycosylation end-products. Excess glucose combines with free amino acids on serum or tissue proteins, initially forming reversible early glycosylation products and later irreversible advanced glycosylation end-products (AGEs). Circulating AGE concentrations are increased in diabetic patients, particularly those with renal insufficiency, because AGEs are normally excreted in the urine. Aminoguanidine, an inhibitor of AGEs, has been shown to diminish proteinuria, mesangial matrix expansion, and basement membrane thickness in diabetic animals. Unfortunately, this drug was found to be too toxic for human use. AGEs increase vascular permeability, promote the influx of mononuclear cells, and stimulate cell proliferation. There is also evidence that AGEs modify low-density lipoprotein (LDL), making it less able to be cleared by the LDL receptors. Thus, AGEs may contribute to the hyperlipidemia commonly present in diabetic patients.

  B. Sorbitol pathway. Glucose that enters cells is metabolized in part via the enzyme aldose reductase. This process is more pronounced with chronic hyperglycemia. The accumulation of sorbitol within the cells leads to a rise in intracellular osmolality and a decrease in intracellular myoinositol, both of which can interfere with cell metabolism. Hyperglycemia may also contribute directly to the decline in cell myoinositol levels by competitively interfering with myoinositol uptake from the extracellular fluid via a sodium–myoinositol co-transporter. The best evidence for sorbitol being a major factor in the etiology of complications is when aldose reductase inhibitors are used to retard cataract formation in animals. Trials in human diabetes have been minimal at best, and the drugs tested to date have been quite toxic.

C.   Protein kinase C. Activation of isomers of protein kinase C (PKC) activity also appears to be an important component of microvascular complications. This increase in activation appears to be caused by enhanced synthesis of diacylglycerol, a major endogenous activator of PKC. Currently, PKC inhibitors are being tested for a variety of vascular complications, including diabetic retinopathy (DR).

II.   Diabetic retinopathy

A.   Prevalence. After 15 years of type 1 diabetes, 80% of patients have some degree of DR, whereas 25% of patients have proliferative DR, the most sight-threatening form of the disease. Slightly fewer patients with type 2 diabetes develop DR, but because of the much larger number of patients with this form of diabetes, many more people with type 2 diabetes have DR. Approximately 5% of all patients with diabetes progress to severe visual loss of 5/200 or more. The major risk factors are glycemic control (best to be thought of as *glycemic exposure*) and hypertension. It is important to appreciate that DR is asymptomatic until the disease has progressed to its late stages.

B.   Classification

1.   Nonproliferative DR. Nonproliferative DR (NPDR) is characterized by structural abnormalities of the retinal vessels, varying degrees of retinal hypoperfusion, retinal edema, lipid exudates, and intraretinal hemorrhages. NPDR may cause visual loss by clinically significant macular edema. Viewing the macula stereoscopically is the only way this can be appreciated.

2.   Proliferative diabetic retinopathy. Neovascularization is the hallmark of proliferative DR. It may occur on the optic disc, elsewhere on the retina, or on the iris (rubeosis iridis). Neovascular tissue contains both a vascular and a fibrous component. The former may cause preretinal or vitreous hemorrhage, whereas the latter may interact with the vitreous to produce traction on the retina and subsequent retinal detachment.

C.   Prevention. It is clear that both blood glucose control and blood pressure control can decrease the risk of the development and progression of DR.

D.   Screening. Recommendations include a yearly dilated retinal examination for individuals with type 2 diabetes. For those with type 1 diabetes, yearly screening examinations should begin after 5 years of disease but not before puberty. Women with diabetes who become pregnant should have a dilated eye examination in the first trimester of pregnancy and close follow-up throughout the pregnancy. Screening examinations should be performed by a trained eye care professional and should include a stereoscopic examination.

E. Treatment. The Diabetic Retinopathy Study showed the effectiveness of panretinal photocoagulation to decrease the likelihood visual acuity will decrease. Furthermore, other studies have shown the effectiveness of focal laser to improve the risk of clinically significant macular edema progressing to severe visual loss. Vitrectomy has also been shown to be effective for severe bleeding into the vitreous. The Early Treatment of Diabetic Retinopathy Study showed that aspirin neither improved nor worsened DR.

F. Rapid improvements in hemoglobin A1c. It needs to be appreciated that a rapid improvement in blood glucose control may cause a worsening of previous DR. Those at highest risk are those with long time periods of poor control [especially with a hemoglobin A1c (A1c) value of >10%] and a moderately advanced stage of NPDR. Although not formally studied, most recommend slow improvement of glucose control in this population with more frequent ophthalmologic evaluations.

G. Other ocular complications. Although not microvascular complications of diabetes, there are other important complications more often seen in patients with diabetes. The first is cataract formation, which is present in 22% of adults with diabetes compared with 3% of those without. For those diagnosed with diabetes after reaching the age of 30 years, cataract formation is responsible for more decrease in vision than DR. Similarly, glaucoma is more common, being present in 7% of individuals with diabetes compared with 1% of the general population. Glycemic control appears to be important for these complications as well.

III. Diabetic nephropathy. Diabetic nephropathy occurs with an overall prevalence of approximately 20% to 30%. Although it is often noted that nephropathy is more common in type 1 than in type 2 diabetes, this point is now under some debate. Younger patients with type 1 diabetes frequently develop end-stage renal disease (ESRD) without significant cardiac disease. On the other hand, older individuals with type 2 diabetes may have significant nephropathy (manifested by heavy proteinuria) with normal renal function when they succumb to coronary artery disease. Proteinuria is an independent risk factor of cardiac death, and these older patients have other risks such as dyslipidemia and hypertension. Furthermore, diabetic nephropathy is more common in certain ethnic populations (African Americans, Native Americans, Mexican Americans) for which the prevalence of type 2 diabetes is increasing. Individuals with type 2 diabetes are the largest group entering treatment programs for ESRD in the United States. The mean 5-year life expectancy for patients with diabetes-related ESRD is <20% in the absence of transplantation.

A. Pathogenesis and pathology. There are three major histologic changes in the glomeruli in diabetic nephropathy: mesangial expansion, glomerular basement membrane thickening, and glomerular sclerosis. These different histologic patterns appear to have similar prognostic significance. The mesangial expansion and glomerulosclerosis do not always develop in parallel, suggesting that they may have somewhat different pathogeneses. Glomerulosclerosis appears to result from intraglomerular hypertension induced by renal vasodilatation or from ischemic injury induced by hyaline narrowing of the vessels supplying the glomeruli. Besides the development of AGEs noted above, activation of cytokines may be another factor involved in the matrix accumulation in diabetic nephropathy. Transforming growth factor-β, for example, may contribute to both the cellular hypertrophy and the enhanced collagen synthesis that are seen in diabetic nephropathy.

B. Albuminuria and proteinuria. The hallmark of diabetic nephropathy is albuminuria, which reflects both histologic and functional abnormalities of the kidney. Microalbuminuria is the earliest laboratory finding in nephropathy and occurs 5 to 8 years before the onset of overt proteinuria. Normoalbuminuria is present with albumin excretion rates below 30 mg per day, whereas microalbuminuria is defined by an albumin excretion rate of 30 to 300 mg per day. An albumin excretion rate of >300 mg per day defines clinical nephropathy, also known as overt proteinuria, dipstick-positive proteinuria, and macroalbuminuria. At this stage, the usual commercial dipstick for proteinuria is positive.

C. Risk factors. Clearly, glycemic control is a major risk factor for diabetic nephropathy. This was shown in both type 1 and type 2 diabetes in the landmark studies the Diabetes Control and Complications Trial and the U.K. Prospective Diabetes Study, respectively. Both of these studies showed an increased risk of developing diabetic nephropathy with increasing levels of A1c. There also is a genetic susceptibility for developing diabetic nephropathy in both type 1 and type 2 diabetes. If one sibling or parent with diabetes has nephropathy, the risk of the diabetic family member developing proteinuria is much higher. Although the exact genetic defect is not known, it may be that the increased risk may be partly found in the angiotensin-converting enzyme

(ACE) gene genotype. Blood pressure is another important risk factor for diabetic nephropathy. In fact, some studies suggest a parental history of hypertension may predispose to diabetic nephropathy. The presence of hypertension does not appear to be as strong a risk factor with improved glycemic control. The risk of nephropathy with a history of hypertension appears to be greatest in patients with the highest levels of A1c (above 12%). Race is another risk factor for diabetic nephropathy. The incidence and severity of diabetic nephropathy are increased in African Americans (three- to sixfold compared with Caucasians), Mexican Americans, and Pima Indians with type 2 diabetes.

D. Relationship between diabetic retinopathy and nephropathy. Patients with type 1 diabetes and diabetic nephropathy almost always have signs on physical exam of DR. However, not everyone with type 1 diabetes and retinopathy will have proteinuria. This relationship is not as predictable for patients with type 2 diabetes.

E. Screening for proteinuria. Current recommendations are screening for proteinuria yearly after 5 years' duration of type 1 diabetes and yearly after the diagnosis of type 2 diabetes (Fig. 7-1). Numerous false positives can occur (Table 7-1), and screening a newly diagnosed patient with type 2 diabetes should be delayed until severe hyperglycemia (average plasma glucose above 300 mg/dL) has been corrected. Initial screen for nephropathy can occur with a standard urine dipstick for proteinuria. A positive reading will detect approximately 500 mg per day of proteinuria, which is equivalent to approximately 300 mg per day of albuminuria. This "dipstick-positive" proteinuria is also termed clinical nephropathy, gross proteinuria, and macroproteinuria. If dipstick-positive proteinuria is found, further screening for a lesser degree of nephropathy (microalbuminuria, defined as 30 to 300 mg per day of albuminuria) is not required. Rather, with this more advanced amount of proteinuria, quantification with a 24-hour urine collection for total proteinuria and creatinine clearance should be performed. Treatment should proceed accordingly (see below). If the dipstick for proteinuria is negative, then screening for microalbuminuria should be performed. There are a variety of acceptable methods for this, including a spot albumin-to-creatinine ratio, a dipstick that measures for microalbuminuria, a timed urine collection for albuminuria (e.g., 4 or 8 hours), and a 24-hour urine collection. If the test is negative, current recommendations are for a repeat measurement in 1 year. If it is

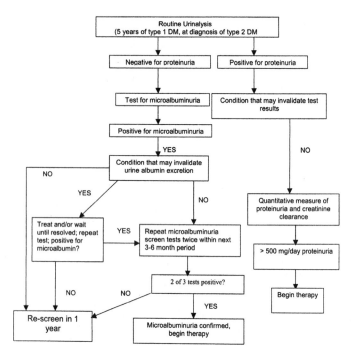

Fig. 7-1. Algorithm for screening for diabetic nephropathy. Screening should be initiated at diagnosis for patients with type 2 diabetes and after 5 years' duration for patients with type 1 diabetes.

positive, it needs to be repeated and shown to be positive before the diagnosis of microalbuminuria can be confirmed. To diagnose microalbuminuria, two of the three screening tests need to be positive. The 24-hour urine collection has a better sensitivity than the other methods, and many clinicians prefer to confirm microalbuminuria with this more sensitive, albeit cumbersome, test.

Table 7-1. Etiologies of false-positive tests for microalbuminuria

Uncontrolled hyperglycemia

Uncontrolled hypertension

Menstrual bleeding

Urinary tract infection

Exercise just prior to or during collection

High-protein diet just prior to collection

Thyrotoxicosis

F.   Treatment of diabetic nephropathy. There are four interventions to consider once albuminuria is discovered.

1.   The first intervention is meticulous glycemic control. Numerous studies have shown that near-normal glucose control can reduce the albumin excretion rate and prevent the progression to overt proteinuria. There are fewer data about the impact of glycemic control with more advanced nephropathy, but available evidence suggests the more advanced the renal disease, the less impact glycemic control will have on slowing its progression.

2.   The second intervention is scrupulous blood pressure control. Studies from the early 1980s clearly showed that controlling systemic blood pressure slows the rate of decline of renal function and improves survival. In these studies, the primary drugs used were cardioselective β-blockers and loop diuretics.

3.   Later, it was shown that ACE inhibitors have an incremental beneficial effect, by virtue of selective efferent arteriolar dilation. Indeed, ACE inhibitors offer beneficial effects on microalbuminuria even in the absence of systemic hypertension. ACE inhibitors also have proven to be of benefit in patients with established nephropathy and mild renal insufficiency. More recently, similar data for patients with diabetic nephropathy have been reported with angiotensin receptor blockers. It has also been shown that blocking the renin–angiotensin system at the level of both the ACE and the angiotensin receptor may be superior than either agent alone.

4.   The fourth intervention for diabetic nephropathy is dietary protein restriction. It is thought that this strategy is useful in reducing renal plasma flow, thus improving glomerular hemodynamics in diabetic renal disease. The American Diabetes Association currently recommends 0.8 g of protein/kg per day (or about 10% of daily total calories) in patients with clinical nephropathy.

IV.   Neuropathy. There are several different classifications of diabetic neuropathy. One such classification is noted in Table 7-2. The two most common neuropathies will be reviewed below.

A.   Painful chronic sensorimotor neuropathy (symmetric polyneuropathy). Painful chronic sensorimotor neuropathy is one of the most common complaints of individuals with diabetes. Estimates vary, but two large studies noted that symptomatic neuropathy had a prevalence of almost 30% in people with diabetes. Another report noted that only 13% of the diabetic pop-

Table 7-2. Classifications of diabetic neuropathy

Peripheral neuropathy
Polyneuropathy
Distal symmetric neuropathy
Sensory loss with numbness
Dysesthesias
Paresthesias
Chronic sensorimotor
Acute sensory
Muscle pain
Neuropathic foot ulceration
Neuroarthropathy (Charcot's joint)
Mononeuropathy
Mononeuropathy
Cranial neuropathies
Compression or entrapment neuropathies
Isolated peripheral
Proximal motor
Mononeuropathy multiplex
Plexopathy
Diabetic truncal neuropathy or radiculopathy
Autonomic neuropathy
Cardiovascular autonomic neuropathy
Cardiac denervation syndrome
Postural hypotension
Gastrointestinal neuropathy
Gastroparesis diabeticorum
Diabetic diarrhea
Fecal incontinence
Constipation
Genitourinary neuropathy
Diabetic cystopathy
Impotence
Female sexual dysfunction
Sudomotor dysfunction
Pupillary abnormalities

ulation had symptomatic neuropathy, yet more than half of the study sample had clinical evidence of neuropathy on examination. Thus, careful clinical examination is important to identify which patients are affected, because an insensate foot is a strong predictor of neuropathic ulcer and lower-extremity amputation. Although decreased vibratory sensation and absent ankle reflexes are the hallmarks of this complication, the inability to appreciate the 10-g (5.07) Semmes–Weinstein monofilament is the simplest and cheapest way to determine if plantar sensation is sufficient to protect from future ulceration. The inability to detect this pressure necessitates further education regarding frequent foot inspection, proper foot care, and the need for extradepth shoes.

 1. Pathogenesis. It is likely that the pathogenesis is multifactorial, with both hyperglycemia and other factors playing a role. Therefore, it is not surprising that there is not a single, definitive treatment to relieve the pain, although improved glycemic control is effective in some patients. Certainly, improving glycemic control can delay progression of neuropathy. There is some suggestion that in addition to improvement of A1c, glycemic stability is also important. Rapid swings from hypoglycemia to hyperglycemia may aggravate neuropathic pain and may actually be more detrimental than continued hyperglycemia.

 2. Treatment. Tricyclic antidepressants have been the first-line drug for the treatment of painful symmetric polyneuropathy. They are not efficacious, however, in everyone, and there is no way to predict whom they will benefit. Some prefer to use amitriptyline for those patients who have difficulty falling asleep. A number of other drugs have been reported to be useful. These include phenytoin, carbamazepine, mexiletine, lidocaine, and topical capsaicin. There has recently been great enthusiasm for the use of gabapentin, and one large clinical trial reported this agent to be beneficial. Unfortunately, there is no mechanism to predict which drug will benefit which patient.

B. Autonomic neuropathy. Autonomic neuropathy is common, but its clinical presentation is quite variable. Parasympathetic dysfunction, which may be manifested only by an increase in heart rate, has been shown to be present in 65% of patients with type 2 diabetes 10 years after diagnosis. One may also document lack of sinus arrhythmia, but there are no data to suggest this should be a routine screening test. Gastroparesis is one of the most frustrating of the autonomic neuropathies. Mild cases can often be treated by the avoidance of high-fat foods in conjunction with either metoclopramide or cisapride. More severe cases can be treated with subcutaneous metoclopramide. Cases presenting with refractory nausea and vomiting often require hospitalization with intravenous metoclopramide. Some patients respond to prochlorperazine, and there are data to suggest that erythromycin, especially if given intravenously, may be effective. Abnormal sweating is another common type of autonomic neuropathy. Gustatory sweating is particularly troublesome, with profuse sweating of the face, trunk, and upper neck associated with eating. More common is reduced sweating of the feet, a form of sympathetic dysfunction. This is potentially a risk factor for plantar fissures and, in combination with sensory polyneuropathy, adds to the risk of a neuropathic ulcer. Moisturizing creams should be used daily in these individuals. One of the most disabling of the autonomic neuropathies is postural hypotension, defined as an orthostatic fall in systolic blood pressure in excess of 20 mm Hg. The mechanism is a combination of central and peripheral cardiovascular sympathetic denervation. Fortunately, it is usually mild, but cases with severe disability, requiring the use of a wheelchair, are not uncommon. Some patients get exacerbations with insulin therapy or with eating. Anemia will also worsen postural hypotension, which is why erythropoietin therapy is effective in patients with advanced renal disease. Treatment can be initiated by discontinuation of aggravating drugs (tricyclics, diuretics). Other general recommendations would include making changes in posture slowly, crossing the legs while actively standing on both legs, and performing dorsiflexion of the feet or handgrip exercise before standing. The mainstay of medical therapy is fludrocortisone (0.1 to 0.4 mg per day) and a high-salt diet. The main side effects of this therapy are hypertension and edema. Alternatives include the α-adrenoreceptor agonist midodrine, the β-blocker pindolol, and fluoxetine. Octreotide may be tried in refractory cases.

SELECTED READING

American Diabetes Association Position Statement. Diabetic nephropathy. *Diabetes Care* 2003;26(suppl 1):94–98.

Bakris GL, Weir M. ACE inhibitors and protection against kidney disease progression in patients with type 2 diabetes: what's the evidence? *J Clin Hypertens* 2002;4:420–423.

Lewis EJ. The role of angiotensin II receptor blockers I preventing the progression of renal disease in patients with type 2 diabetes. *Am J Hypertens* 2002;15:123S–128S.

Ritz E, Orth SR. Nephropathy in patients with type 2 diabetes. *N Engl J Med* 1999;341:1127–1133.

Tobe SW, McFarlane PA, Naimark DM. Microalbuminuria in diabetes mellitus. *Can Med Assoc J* 2002;167:499–503.

Vivian EM, Rubinswtein GB. Pharmacologic management of diabetic nephropathy. *Clin Ther* 2002;24:1741–1756.

Macrovascular Complications

In a survey done in 2001, of approximately 2,000 people with diabetes, 68% of individuals did not consider cardiovascular disease (CVD) to be a serious complication associated with diabetes mellitus in contrast to 65% acknowledging blindness as associated with diabetes. Of these same individuals, 60% did not feel that having diabetes increased the risk of developing hypertension or elevated cholesterol. Yet CVD is the major diabetes-associated complication leading to not only chronic illness but also early mortality. A two- to fourfold increased risk in coronary artery disease with a twofold increase in coronary heart disease (CHD) mortality in men and fivefold increase in women with diabetes are seen. CVD is the underlying cause of death in patients with diabetes, with ischemic heart disease the major contributor in almost two-thirds of these patients, followed by cerebrovascular disease and other heart disease. This has formed the basis of current recommendations that diabetes mellitus be considered an endovascular disease and treated as aggressively as documented CVD in the nondiabetic individual.

I. Long-term mortality comparisons among nondiabetic individuals with previous myocardial infarction (MI), compared with diabetic individuals without previous MI, show essentially the same mortality rate. Additionally, diabetic patients without previous CVD have the same risk of new MI as nondiabetic individuals with CVD after hospitalization for unstable coronary disease. For specific manifestations of CVD such as intermittent claudication in men and heart failure in women, relative risk of an event was five times higher in the diabetic as compared with the nondiabetic subject in the Framingham Heart Study follow-up.

A. The decline in coronary heart disease mortality in the United States over the last 30 years has not been shown in the diabetic population. CHD death rates have decreased 36.4% in nondiabetic men but only

13.1% in men with diabetes. For nondiabetic women, the decrease in CHD mortality of 27% has been accompanied by an increase in mortality of 23% among diabetic women. This increase was observed over an age range of 35 to 74 years but was most pronounced in the younger age group.

B. Thirty percent to 50% of ischemic episodes occur without recognized symptoms in both nondiabetic individuals and patients with diabetes. Electrocardiographic (ECG) evidence of schemia is more common in the diabetic person. In men, silent myocardial schemia, defined as ≥1 mm ST-segment depression on exercise or ambulatory ECG monitoring, has been shown to be associated with autonomic dysfunction of the heart, with defects seen on thallium scan. Further, reduced coronary vasodilation after submaximal increases in myocardial muscle demand might further explain diabetic silent schemia. Which testing modality to use for screening for the prevalence of myocardial schemia remains unclear, but current recommendation is to screen all type 2 diabetic patients with >10 years' known duration or with additional risk factor of CVD disease with Holter monitoring, exercise ECG, or thallium scan.

C. Myocardial infarction has been associated with more extensive coronary atherosclerosis in the diabetic individual, which may limit the efficacy of thrombolytic therapy. The size of an MI is not typically larger in the person with diabetes, although acute arrhythmias, cardiogenic shock, myocardial rupture, and early mortality are more likely. Anterior MI is associated with a higher mortality rate at 60 days in the diabetic versus nondiabetic subject. Recurrent MI is more common in the diabetic woman if concomitant congestive heart failure (CHF) develops. Additional factors increasing post-MI overall mortality are kidney failure and older age as well as glycemic control.

1. Revascularization attempt with angioplasty without stent placement has less success in diabetic than nondiabetic patients, with higher rates of restenosis. More recent studies suggest this difference might not be as marked with stent placement at the time of angioplasty. However, coronary artery bypass grafting compared with percutaneous transluminal coronary angioplasty in the Bypass Angioplasty Revascularization Investigation was associated at 5-year follow-up in diabetic patients with coronary schemia and more than two documented obstructions in major coronary arteries, with lower death rate (19% versus 34%). There was also a reduced death rate after spontaneous

Q-wave MI (relative risk, 0.09%; 95% confidence interval, 0.03 to 0.29). Follow-up data to 7 years from event have continued to show less mortality in the group undergoing coronary artery bypass graft.

2. Congestive heart failure incidence is increased twofold in men with diabetes and fivefold in women with diabetes. Factors felt to contribute to the greater burden of CHF in diabetic subjects include MI size, long-standing hypertension, and microvascular disease with pathologically seen arteriolar thickening, microaneurysms, and basement membrane thickening in diabetic individuals dying of CHF. Diastolic dysfunction may be more common in the diabetic person, with increased left ventricular end-diastolic pressure, reduced left ventricular end-diastolic volume, but normal ejection fraction. A restrictive or dilated cardiomyopathy may be present in diabetic patients with clinical CHF.

3. Conduction disorders such as left bundle branch block and atrial fibrillation are more common in diabetic patients. Cardiac autonomic neuropathy manifesting as increased heart rate at rest, less beat-to-beat variability in heart rhythm, and orthostatic hypotension is associated with lower 5-year survival in the person with diabetes and coronary disease.

II. Risk factors for CVD in the diabetic individual are mostly the same as in the nondiabetic. Smoking, hypertension, dyslipidemia, as well as obesity, sedentary lifestyle, and family history of CVD are shared risk factors. Type 2 diabetes is also specifically associated with alterations in coagulation and fibrinolysis. As it is not clear which of these factors has a primary role, making prioritization difficult, it is felt that attention to all, as well as to maximally controlling hyperglycemia, should be targeted.

A. The role of glycemic control in the prevention of CHD remains unclear. Although statistical significance has not been reached, trends toward less cardiovascular burden with improved glycemic control have been observed. In the Diabetes Control and Complications Trial involving type 1 diabetes, the design was to look at intensive glucose control in relation to the impact of developing microvascular disease. Improved lipid levels, lower blood pressure, and lower macrovascular complications were seen in the intensive treatment cohort, but the 42% reduction in cardiovascular events was not statistically significant ($p = 0.065$). The small number of events observed, however, limits the interpretation of these data. In type 2 diabetes, the U.K. Prospective Diabetes Study (UKPDS) showed a trend toward less fatal and nonfatal MI with a 16% reduction in events in the intensively controlled, but statistically this just missed significance ($p = 0.052$). Observational data do suggest benefit, but it is difficult to assess glycemic benefit without also taking into consideration benefit of improved glycemic control on improved lipid fractions, cytokines, and other CVD-associated risk factors. However, it is clear that improved glucose control is associated with less cardiovascular morbidity and mortality when treated in the intensive care unit and coronary care unit patient, so improving glycemic control should remain a part of CVD prevention strategy, both for primary as well as for secondary intervention. Among oral agents, metformin has shown particular benefit as compared with sulfonylurea treatment in the UKPDS.

B.   Hypertension affects 20% to 60% of people with diabetes, depending on age, body mass index, and ethnicity. In type 1 diabetes, hypertension is frequently associated with existing renal insufficiency. In type 2, it is often associated in combination with obesity and dyslipidemia, as part of the dysmetabolic syndrome. Epidemiologic trials suggest an increased cardiovascular event rate with values over 120 mm Hg systolic and 80 mm Hg diastolic. Randomized control trials, including the UKPDS, support the benefit of lowering blood pressure to at least <140/80 mm Hg. Current American Diabetes Association guidelines suggest ≤130/80 mm Hg as target level, based primarily on the Hypertension Optimal Trial (HOT), in which a targeted diastolic pressure of <80 mm Hg was associated with a 50% decrease in fatal and nonfatal MI, stroke, and cardiovascular death.

1.   Various prospective studies have shown a **number of antihypertensive agents** to be beneficial in reducing hypertension and reducing CHD events in type 2 diabetes. The Systolic Hypertension in the Elderly, Systolic Hypertension in Europe, HOT, and UKPDS all showed reduced CHD events with hypertension agents of various classes. Angiotensin-converting inhibitor therapy has most consistently been shown to have the most therapeutic impact in an analysis of several trials including the Appropriate Blood Pressure Control in Diabetes (ABCD) comparing enalapril with nisoldipine, the Captopril Prevention Project (CAPP) comparing captopril with β-androgen blockers or diuretics, the Fosinopril versus Amlodipine Cardiovascular Events Trial (FACET) comparing fosinopril and amlodipine, and the UKPDS comparing captopril with atenolol. ABCD, CAPP, and FACET all showed significant benefit of angiotensin-converting enzyme (ACE) therapy over the others tried, in decreased MI events, other CVD events, and all-cause mortality. The Heart Outcomes Prevention Evaluation Study (HOPE) further showed the benefit of ACE inhibitor therapy using ramipril (although not as an antihypertensive, as blood pressure was lowered only by 2/1 mm Hg in the treated group) in decreasing MI, CVD, and stroke events. This effect was even more pronounced in the Microalbuminuria, Cardiovascular, and Renal Outcomes subset of HOPE. Only in the UKPDS was there no clear benefit when comparing ACE with β-blocker, which has raised the issue as to which of these two agents is preferred. However, given that ACE inhibitors are also renoprotective and possibly afford retinal protective effect, they are the preferred treatment class of antihypertensive. Recently, angiotensin receptor blockers (ARBs) have also been shown to be effective as antihypertensive agents with decreased cardiovascular event rate and can be used as first-line blood pressure therapy or as alternate therapy when cough prevents use of ACE.

2. In the setting of microalbuminuria, angiotensin-converting enzyme or angiotensin receptor blocker is preferred. In patients with recent MI, β-blockers have been shown to reduce postevent mortality and should be considered as additional therapy to ACE or ARB. α-Blockers were shown to be considerable less effective drugs than diuretics in reducing CHF in the Antihypertensive and Lipid-Lowering Treatment to Prevent Heart Attack Trial and continue to be considered third- or fourth-line antihypertensives. Most diabetic patients will require more than monotherapy to achieve target blood pressure control. Combination of ACE and/or ARB with a diuretic can be effective, followed by a nondihydropyridine calcium channel blocker. When starting ACE or ARB, potassium should be monitored closely as well as creatinine. A slight creatinine rise can often be seen with ACE or ARB initiation and is not reason for drug discontinuance unless creatinine continues to rise.

C. Lipid lowering has been shown in several trials to decrease the incidence of cardiovascular events in diabetic subjects. Secondary prevention trials using the statin agents simvastatin and pravastatin have shown in diabetic subpopulations a greater therapeutic benefit than in the nondiabetic, although actual diabetic patient numbers were small and generally serum low-density lipoprotein (LDL) cholesterol is only slightly, if at all, elevated. In the Scandinavian Simvastatin Survival Study, a 34% reduction in LDL-cholesterol, with triglyceride decrease of 11% and high-density lipoprotein (HDL) increase of 7%, similar to that seen in the treated nondiabetic population, resulted in a 75% decreased probability of a major CHD event over 6 years as compared with 51% in placebo-treated patients. This translated to a 55% reduction in risk in the treated diabetic patient as compared with the treated nondiabetic patient. In the Cholesterol and Recurrent Events Trial, pravastatin reduced the relative risk of coronary events by 25% in diabetic patients ($p < 0.05$) and 23% in nondiabetic subjects ($p < 0.001$). Among 4,000 individuals with diabetes enrolled in the Heart Protection Study receiving 40 mg of simvastatin, there was a 25% reduction in major CVD event, even in those with LDL at ≤116 mg/dL, irrespective of a prior CHD event, hypertension, age, or gender, suggesting no threshold in LDL effect. Other lipid profile subfractions are also important, as shown in the Helsinki Heart Study, with the use of gemfibrozil to decrease triglycerides and increase HDL-cholesterol, and the Veterans Affairs Cooperative Studies Program High-Density Lipoprotein Cholesterol Intervention Trial, also using gemfibrozil. The LDL reduction was minimal, but a 22% reduction in CHD death and nonfatal MI ($p = 0.006$) was seen. Prospectively, fenofibrate in the Diabetes Atherosclerosis Intervention Study reduced stenosis over 3 years, although the study was not powered to look at whether this translated to event reduction.

1. Although improved glycemic control could favorably impact on lipid profile as well as lifestyle change with increased physical activity and medical nutrition therapy, for most individuals, pharmacotherapy will be needed to treat lipids to current goals of LDL-cholesterol level of ≤100 mg/dL, triglycerides of ≤150 mg/dL, and HDL-cholesterol of ≥40 mg/dL.

2. Statins remain the therapy of choice for LDL lowering, and both simvastatin and atorvastatin can additionally increase HDL and lower triglycerides, although modestly. Statins are generally well tolerated: In the Heart Protection Study, a cohort of over 20,000 individuals aged 40 to 80 years had an annual excess risk of myopathy of 0.01% when statins were used at a compliance rate of 80%. If triglycerides are targeted for therapy, fibric acid derivatives are the drugs of choice. Niacin is best to increase HDL but may have dose limitations with regard to both its potential in raising glucose and tolerance to side effects of flush-

ing. Slow-release forms of niacin can be easier to tolerate and might be more likely to increase glucose only transiently. Niacin also can decrease Lp(a), although there is still disagreement about a measurement standard for Lp(a), making it difficult to know its clear role in diabetic CHD risk. Although a combination niacin and statin product is on the market, liver function should be monitored at least twice a year if either this combination or a combined fibric acid and statin combination are used. Frail, older women taking other medications seem to be at particular risk to develop a myositis while taking a fibric acid derivative with statin. Drugs such as macrolide antibiotics, cyclosporine, and certain antifungals affect hepatic clearance of statins and therefore can lead to increased toxicity when used concurrently. Creatine kinase (CPK) level exceeding three to four times the upper level of normal in the setting of symptoms warrants drug discontinuance, although even a trend of increasing CPK should be viewed as a potential reason to drop one agent. Unfortunately, although CPK screening can be helpful, it will not always be elevated in the presence of symptoms, so clinical judgment in the setting of muscle symptoms should be exercised. Combination of just-released ezetimide with a statin can increase LDL lowering by an additional 20% to 40%. Ezetimide is a new class of cholesterol-lowering agent acting at the intestinal brush border. Its efficacy specifically in diabetic patients needs further study.

D. Lifestyle modification is difficult to achieve but remains a cornerstone to decreasing CHD event risk. It often tends to be overlooked or deliberately ignored as increasingly pharmacotherapy is seen as more successful and more favorable in provider time cost/benefit ratio.

1. Weight management and physical activity in particular have been shown to be associated with decreased CHD. Setting short-term practical goals is helpful and can impact quickly on glycemic measures, triglyceride levels, and hypertension control. Emphasizing complex carbohydrate intake over simple carbohydrates, embodied in the concept of glycemic index, has been shown in small studies to reduce triglycerides and raise HDL-cholesterol. Hidden sources of excess calories such as 6 oz of red wine, which contains 120 cal (as much as a 12-oz can of regular soda), can accumulate quickly, if not ingested in moderation. Skipping desserts when eating out, splitting a main entree, and substituting monounsaturated fatty acids and n-3 polyunsaturated fatty acids for saturated fatty acids, such as tree nuts and avocados for hot dogs and bacon, can improve lipid levels, decrease insulin resistance, improve platelet function, as well as decrease blood pressure. Decreasing fast food intake frequency to once a week or less, taking the stairs rather than elevator even if for one flight, and parking at some distance from building entry are simple recommendations that have been shown to be more effective if written out on a prescription pad. Reduction in intra-abdominal fat in particular is associated with decreased insulin resistance.

   2.   Cigarette smoking increased the relative risk of CVD twofold in diabetics in the Multiple Risk Factor Intervention Trial (MRFIT).

   3. Although **alcohol consumption** has been shown to reduce CVD risk by 50% to 60% in diabetic patients in prospective studies, its contribution to total caloric intake, its potential appetite-stimulatory effect, and the potential for significant hypoglycemia suggest its use should be limited.

   E.   Coagulation abnormalities in patients with insulin resistance increase the risk of accelerated atherosclerosis and thrombosis. Decreased tissue plasminogen activator activity, decreased α_2-antitrypsin, and increased levels of plasminogen activator inhibitor reduce fibrinolysis, whereas platelet hyperaggregability and increased levels of procoagulants favor clot formation. Aspirin induces a protective effect through blocking thromboxane activity and acetylating platelet cyclooxygenase. Dosages in trials have ranged from 75 to 325 mg per day, and benefits have been seen across age ranges, genders, and both the presence and the absence of previous CVD or hypertension. Use in patients below the age of 21 years can be associated with Reye's syndrome. ACE inhibitors have been shown to reduce plasminogen activator inhibitor-1 activity and antigen levels in patients. This may provide another explanation of the benefits of ACE inhibitors independent of blood pressure–lowering effects. Although aspirin was thought to potentially lessen the benefits of ACE inhibitors in patients with established CVD, this has not been shown in more recent analyses.

SELECTED READING

American Diabetes Association. Standards of medical care for patients with diabetes mellitus. *Diabetes Care* 2002;25:213–229.

Heart Protection Study Collaborative Group. MRC/BHF Heart Protection Study of cholesterol lowering with simvastatin in 20,536 high-risk individuals: a randomised placebo-controlled study. *Lancet* 2002;360:7–22.

Kaplan NM. Management of hypertension in patients with type 2 diabetes mellitus: guidelines based on current evidence. *Ann Intern Med* 2001;135:1079–1083.

O'Keefe JH, Wetzel M, Moe RR, et al. Should an angiotensin-converting enzyme inhibitor be standard therapy for patients with atherosclerotic disease? *J Am Coll Cardiol* 2001;37:1–8.

Sobel BE. Potentiation of vasculopathy by insulin. Implications from an NHLBI clinical alert. *Circulation* 1996;93:1613–1615.

Wilson PWF. Diabetes mellitus and coronary heart disease. *Endocrinol Clin North Am* 2001;30:857–881.

Psychosocial Issues

Diabetes is unique as a chronic disease in its association with changes in emotional well-being that can have profound effects in turn on the cognitive challenges of the maintenance of the disease itself. When compared with other illnesses such as asthma, rheumatoid arthritis, or even oncologic illness, the prevalence of depression is greater in the diabetic individual. Specific subpopulations with diabetes have additional confounding factors: Women with type 1 diabetes have a higher prevalence of eating disorders, and older people with type 2 diabetes have an associated alteration in cognitive function often affecting memory or problem-solving capability. Specific ethnic populations have cultural beliefs that might affect not just acceptance of the diagnosis of diabetes but also acceptance of specific treatment modalities.

I. Barriers to self-care include attitudes that might be preformed on the basis of previous experience with others, family, friends, or co-workers, having the diagnosis of diabetes. As an example, in African American culture, the frequently seen associated co-morbidities of diabetes have led to the beliefs that diabetes is associated with early mortality and that there is no way that the natural course of diabetes can be altered to avoid the co-morbidities of limb loss, vision loss, etc. Consequently, having the diagnosis made of diabetes is then likened to being told that death is imminent.

A. Among Hmong populations, the decision to start insulin may need to be made by the family unit, not by the individual affected.

B. In the Ojibway–Cree of northern Ontario, perceptions of the significance of food choice in the development of diabetes and the lack of perception regarding the benefit of physical exercise are being used to target treatment modalities specific to the choice of traditional Indian foods and the limit or avoidance of simple carbohydrates and soda, with much less focus on physical activity as a component of diabetes treatment.

C. Challenges of family members caring for frail American Indian elders with diabetes include anxiety about in-home care, decision-making and communication problems with other family members, and the importance of developing a care routine for successful diabetes management.

II. **Stages of diabetes** may be used as a method to categorize the specific psychosocial challenges of diabetes, specifically diagnosis and initial management, the routine in prevention of medical complications, the onset of complications, and dealing with complications. Alternatively, these can also be divided into specific challenges in dealing with preadolescents, adolescents, the middle-aged, and the elderly. For this section, the former categorization will be used.

    A. **Onset of diabetes** for the type 1 patient is typically very abrupt, resulting in the need for sudden and very significant lifestyle changes. Learning insulin pharmacology and injection skills for survival is complemented by need to learn a wide range of new information regarding diet, interaction between medication and physical activity, and self-blood glucose monitoring. All stages of acceptance will be seen, from mourning and sense of loss of previous freedom in lifestyle and of health by the patient and family to shock and denial of the diagnosis and its implications. The degree to which each of these emotions takes place can be tempered by previous patient and/or family experience with diabetes, as complications of diabetes are envisioned for the newly diagnosed individual. Moving from the acknowledgment stage—that "I am ill"—to an adaptive stage that allows for the learning of demanding and often complex therapy to prevent future end-organ complications needs to be guided by first improving the patient's sense of current well-being. Positive role models can be helpful, from public figures in sports, entertainment, or other popular venues, particularly in helping the child and adolescent deal with the new diabetes diagnosis. Community resources including support groups and diabetes camps can additionally be helpful in giving the younger patient a sense of belonging and a feeling of not being isolated with the management challenges of diabetes. Increasingly, emphasis is now being placed on the importance of even young children assuming some responsibility for self-care such as injecting predrawn insulin themselves, performing self blood glucose monitoring, and even making dietary choices, where knowledge and comfort are present. In type 2 diabetes, which now is increasingly seen in younger individuals, the need to take a pill may not be seen as different from taking a supplement or a prescribed medication. However, use of insulin still has a powerful

illness connotation, a sense of a more serious illness
that may result in a rather abrupt transition of awareness that the diabetes is, indeed, now serious, whereas
previously it was more a nuisance or life-adaptive factor
in the same category as taking a pill for hypertension or
dyslipidemia. Further affecting the psychosocial issues
of the early diagnosis of diabetes is the attitude of the
health care team, the relationship that the patient or
family may have previously had with their health care
provider, as well as the financial support that the patient or family have regarding insurance coverage versus direct out-of-pocket expenses.

B. The routine of diabetes management revolves
around the acceptance of task performance for eventual
benefit that might be viewed as quite distant, if not re-
mote in the future. There is a sense of new identity ac-
quisition and of a need for greater regularization of
habits relating to very basic factors such as eating, always carrying food along to treat possible hypoglycemia, and carrying self-testing equipment. Even the
stigma of a syringe can be denial provoking, particularly in school situations where students often have to
leave the classroom to test their blood. Schools typically
require students to obtain permission to treat symptoms of hypoglycemia that in a personal setting, such as
home, could be attended to more rapidly and with much
less intrusive attention, especially for drawing up and
injecting insulin—actions that, at home, might be done
routinely. In studies of children and their families, although emotional distress can be experienced initially,
decreased self-esteem and increased psychopathology
have not been shown. Yet even adults struggle with insulin injection in public places, even public restrooms,
with the connotation of chemical abuse. In adolescence,
depression may not be evident as patients struggle to
cope with diabetes at the same time as they cope with
their personal identity as they transition from child to
adult. College students with newly acquired indepen-
dence and erratic schedules can also be a challenging
population to guide in self-management of diabetes. Issues that have evolved from focus groups on the challenges and barriers to care in this specific population include the need to address convenient ways to manage
diabetes (such as use of rapid 5-minute turnaround
time for finger-stick glucose readout), motivators to
manage diabetes (e.g., less fatigue, less likelihood of hypoglycemia or hyperglycemic fluctuations), and social
support (such as guidance in managing perceived dietary restrictions, alcohol intake when using insulin). A
health care team versed in issues of not only adoles-

cence but also diabetes is important to provide the support needed in this younger population. For the adult, the more immediate change in lifestyle is frequently followed by an experimental stage in which increasingly old habits are resumed or a sense of challenge to the new lifestyle comes into play.

Foods are used to test the limits of pharmacologic intervention, and a decrease in self-blood glucose monitoring due to a sense that "I can feel my glucose and therefore do not need to test" may become evident. To some extent, this experimentation may be positive in helping the patient and the provider establish a compromise in areas such as glucose testing that otherwise might be mitigated by undisclosed issues such as financial concerns. However, continued follow-up and medical team contact are important for discussing the outcome of patient behavior change.

C. **The onset of complications** typically initiates a sense of anxiety that might include guilt at not following previous medical recommendations for diabetes management and even fear of the meaning of even the slightest finding associated with potential end-organ damage. Mild background retinopathy, the first report of microalbuminuria, and decreased sensation on monofilament challenge can be viewed as harbingers of a cascade of loss. Ophthalmology visits, in particular, are viewed as frightening owing to fear of blindness, but this anxiety escalates when patients are told that eye ground changes, however mild, are seen. Thus, when screening procedures are recommended, however routine they may seem to the clinician, they need to be explained in a preventative light. If tests are indeed positive, it is useful to ask patients how they interpret the news: Benchmarks of family or friends having experience of a complication will be used by patients as a guide to their own future experience and so need to be addressed in the light of current medical knowledge and practice. Consultation with specialists can be very helpful to patients at this time, particularly with an endocrinologist, to help formulate diabetes management as well as provide information as to expectations of potential complication development. Often depression can form a barrier to preventing the very progression of the complication that the patient is worried about. Treatment for depression should be started promptly and efficacy of therapy reviewed frequently, with psychology or psychiatry consultation as indicated. Complications that might be embarrassing for the patient to mention, such as erectile dysfunction, should also be periodically addressed through questioning; this may play a critical role in treating the anxiety as well as fear associated with frequent misconceptions of the significance and treatment of symptoms. Alcohol and other chemical or supplement use should be questioned, which could potentially add to depression or contribute to the complication investigated.

D.   Significant co-morbid conditions begin a stage in which the condition itself starts to require regular medical care and treatment. End-stage renal failure and laser therapy for proliferative retinopathy are examples of conditions in which patients not only has to care for their diabetes but now also have an additional burden of care for another illness. Depression is common, along with a sense of anxiety and fear about the perceived finiteness of life. Alternatively, there can be a sense of elation and expectation of cure in anticipating, for example, a renal transplant, which can lead to profound disappointment when the outcome does not match the expectation.

III.   Behavioral issues pertaining to diabetes are thought to contribute to depression in type 1, with evidence supporting subtle decrements in cognitive function in type 1 diabetes diagnosed before age 5 years and in older type 2 patients. Hypoglycemia in the Diabetes Complications and Control Trial was not associated with change in cognitive function. However, postulated hyper- and hypoglycemia have been speculated potentially to affect areas of the brain that regulate affect. Frequently associated eating disorders as well as anxiety and even guilt could be further contributing factors. The patient–provider relationship is the centerpiece of care, although, when possible, this should be a team joining patient with providers encompassing physician, nurse educator, registered dietitian, pharmacist, psychologist, and others as needed. A sense of collaboration with the patient can build a structured yet open relationship that allows for needed target therapeutic interventions yet also an open atmosphere for the patient to frankly discuss concerns outside immediate laboratory or complication screening guidelines. Differences between patient and clinician goals should be negotiated. Energy needed to deal with family or work issues, such as pending divorce or recent loss of job, may not afford energy to deal with the goal of more frequent glucose monitoring. Patients might at times need support in taking a "diabetes holiday" in which self-monitoring frequency is significantly tapered back for a week or more, or medical nutrition therapy might have to be loosened. Listening to the patient is critical to the success of any treatment program and, although obvious, is often forgotten in an era of provider regulations of numerical goal attainment as a measurement of practice success.

IV.   Identification and treatment of common psychologic disorders in diabetes is within the realm of the primary care provider. Depression, in particular, should be recognized and treated, as in diabetic individuals there is evidence to suggest increased likelihood of recurrent depression even if a single episode of depression remits. Screening for other endocrinopathies should also be done, particularly for thyroid, parathyroid, and less commonly adrenal disorder, as these disorders can result in a depression that can be indistinguishable from primary depressive disorder. Poorly controlled diabetes can present with fatigue, loss of energy, loss of interest or pleasure, and social withdrawal. Also difficult to distinguish from depression, unless noted, are guilt, pessimism, and suicidal ideation. Eating disorders including purging, vomiting, laxative use, and insulin underdosing are more difficult to diagnose, as this is behavior that is hidden and will rarely be shared by the patient, even with the most nonjudgmental questioning. Although a frequent etiology of hospital admission for diabetic ketoacidosis in the female adolescent with diabetes, it can be seen in subtle forms in females and males of all ages, in a society stigmatizing weight.

A. Choice of medication for the treatment of depression in diabetic individuals needs awareness of potential side effects. Older tricyclics have been associated with hyperglycemia, and all have risk of cardiac arrhythmia in the presence of co-existing cardiac disease. Selective serotonin reuptake inhibitors (SSRIs) are associated with potential erectile dysfunction and possible aggravation of gastroparesis (although they can also be therapeutic for gastroparesis).

B. Dosing of any agent should be titrated to achieve maximum effect. This requires monitoring of symptoms. The patient needs to have frequent and regular follow-up.

C. Frequently, monotherapy will not be sufficient for full therapeutic response. As example, the SSRIs might need to be prescribed with a sedative, hypnotic, or sedating antidepressant if insomnia is part of the depression symptom complex. Trazodone is commonly prescribed for this purpose in conjunction with the SSRI.

D. Treatment should be maintained over 4 to 6 months, even for an initial depressive episode. Titration of medication may require several weeks to achieve maximal efficacy. Cognitive behavioral therapy can be an effective adjunct to pharmacotherapy, as this therapy can focus on feelings accompanying depression, such as pessimism, which, when addressed, might allow for not only more successful outcome but also decreased long-term antidepressant therapy need.

E.   Pharmacologic intervention can also be used in eating disorder treatment. Associated depressive disorders can be treated with antidepressants, and for serious cognitive distortions related to body image, respiradone has been used. Group setting and involvement of family are parts of the social psychological behavioral therapy used as a mainstay of eating disorder therapy. Reinstitution of insulin at therapeutic doses can be associated with significant emotional decompensation due to weight gain primarily from initial fluid shift. Hospitalization might be required for monitoring specifically to prevent renewed attempts at purging.

V.   Psychoeducational intervention has come to be used more as a tool for teaching coping skills for particularly intensive and rigorous diabetes treatment programs. These have included blood glucose awareness training with specific attention to hypoglycemia symptom awareness and appropriate treatment through use of detailed diary logs of glucose levels, symptoms, and food intake; coping skills training using role playing and vignettes, particularly in aiding adolescents deal with diabetes treatment regimens; and cognitive behavior treatment programs to help manage stress, aid in personal goal setting, and examine beliefs as barriers to optimizing care.

SELECTED READING

Delamater AM, Jacobson AM, Anderson B, et al. Psychosocial therapies in diabetes: report of the Psychosocial Therapies Working Group. *Diabetes Care* 2001;24:1286–1292.

Grey M, Boland EA, Yu C, et al. Personal and family factors associated with quality of life in adolescents with diabetes. *Diabetes Care* 1998;21:909–914.

Jacobson AM, Weinger K. Psychosocial complications of diabetes. In: Leahy JL, Clark NC, Cefalu WT, eds. *Medical management of diabetes mellitus.* New York: Marcel Dekker, 2000:559–572.

Rose M, Fliege H, Hildebrandt M, et al. The network of psychological variables in patients with diabetes and their importance for quality of life and metabolic control. *Diabetes Care* 2002;25: 35–42.

Samuel–Hodge CD, Headen SW, Skelly AH, et al. Influences on day-to-day self-management of type 2 diabetes among African–American women. *Diabetes Care* 2000;23:928–933.

Surwit RS, van Tilburg MAL, Zucker N, et al. Stress management improves long-term glycemic control in type 2 diabetes. *Diabetes Care* 2002;25:30–34.

Women and Diabetes

Diabetes affects women uniquely. These effects can be divided into specific stages of life: adolescence, reproductive years, menopause, and fragile elderly. Although much remains unclear, as observational studies versus randomized, prospective studies have so recently shown, increasing information about specific conditions affecting women with diabetes or increased risk for development of diabetes has grown in past years.

I. Adolescence concerns have included increased recognition of polycystic ovarian syndrome (PCOS) and its significant risk for development of diabetes mellitus. PCOS is indeed a syndrome, defined by the combination of menstrual irregularity (anovulatory cycles) with biochemical evidence of the presence of more male-like hormone than normal. The finding of cysts on or in the ovary by ultrasound may be referred to as polycystic ovaries, but the PCOS is a metabolic abnormality that does not require ultrasound presence of cysts. Ultrasound of the ovaries done in large numbers of women has shown up to 21% to 22% can have polycystic ovaries. It is estimated that PCOS occurs in about 5% of all women. Depending on the ethnicity of the examined population, prevalence can vary from 3.5% to 11.2% of females.

A. Symptoms of polycystic ovarian syndrome include menstrual irregularity as the hallmark. Periods are infrequent, occurring typically less than six times per year, or may be completely absent. Bleeding at times of menses can vary from spotting to substantial flow. There are few symptoms heralding menses onset as ovulation is absent. Although menstrual irregularity can be present in the first 1 to 1.5 years following menarche, in the adolescent with PCOS, this irregularity will persist. Spontaneous pregnancy rarely occurs, and there may be an increased risk of pregnancy loss when pregnancy does occur. Clinical evidence of excess androgen effect is seen by increased hair growth, particularly on the face and chin, but can also be seen on the lower abdominal wall, chest, and back. Hair thinning or loss can be seen on the scalp. Acne may be present. Acanthosis nigricans can be observed at the base of the back of the neck, in axillary areas, and at the waist. Fifty percent of women with PCOS are obese, with "apple"-type body form, with waist measurement as compared with hip in a higher than normal ratio.

  B.   Diagnosis is made by documenting medical history of menstrual irregularity and obtaining laboratory data of excess androgen presence. Physical exam should look for signs of androgen excess, and weight and blood pressure should be noted. Laboratory testing should include testosterone, androstenedione, and dehydroepiandrostenedione sulfate. There is a characteristic increase in luteinizing hormone as compared with follicle-stimulating hormone in about two-thirds of women with PCOS. Controversy exists over the best way to document insulin resistance: Oral glucose tolerance testing will support the diagnosis of prediabetes or diabetes, but whether a random or a fasting glucose-to-insulin ratio is helpful remains unclear. A lipid profile should include triglycerides and cholesterol subfractions of high-density (HDL) and low-density lipoprotein.

    1.   Differential diagnosis includes the adult variant of congenital adrenal hyperplasia, Cushing's syndrome, and idiopathic hyperandrogenicity. Laboratory testing can be helpful in the differentiation through adrenocorticotrophic hormone–stimulated 12-hydroxyprogesterone levels and dexamethasone suppression testing for cortisol.

    2.   The specific cause of polycystic ovarian syndrome is unclear, although there is known genetic linkage, with typically a positive family history of PCOS and/or type 2 diabetes.

  C.   Treatment goals can vary, depending on individual concerns such as to whether pregnancy is desired, body hair is cosmetically problematic, or weight management is a goal. It is not clear whether there is an optimal frequency of menses per year that is associated with an optimal estrogen effect or a decreased androgen effect that would have maximal benefit regarding bone density, cardiovascular health, or other estrogen-associated benefits. Clearly, these estrogen-related benefits need prospective study evaluation as to their true efficacy, as shown in the difference recently between observational and randomized control trial results in the Women's Health Initiative.

    1.   To induce menses, low-androgen progesterone oral contraceptives or metformin can be used. There are anecdotal reports of currently available thiazolidinediones also inducing ovulation and pregnancy, although metformin has been studied the most thoroughly of the insulin sensitizers, with an estimated ovulation induction success rate of 60%. The effective dose of metformin can vary from 500 up to 2,000 mg per day. It can be slowly titrated in monthly increments (see Chapter 5) both to minimize side effects as well as to evaluate therapeutic efficacy. Antiandrogen treatments such as spironolactone are often also added to achieve maximal therapy benefit. The addition of metformin to oral contraceptive might decrease potential weight gain that can be seen with the oral contraceptive alone.

2.   Spironolactone can be used to treat hirsutism, although oral contraceptives can also be effective. Spironolactone has both estrogen-like and mild anti-androgen-like effects but may take up to 6 months for any significant change in body hair to be appreciated, and up to a year for full effect. Other medications tried include anti-androgens such as finasteride and flutamide. A new topical agent called Vaniqa (eflornithine HCl) might be helpful for facial hair treatment, but as yet reports of effects specific to women with PCOS are not available. A powerful, although difficult-to-achieve, treatment is weight loss.

3.   Metformin was associated with weight loss in some studies, and it has been questioned whether this weight loss alone might be the reason for the medication's beneficial effects in PCOS. It is clear that however achieved, weight loss can reverse many of the effects of PCOS from anovulation to decreased risk of prediabetes and diabetes. Practical lifestyle change recommendations will be reviewed in Chapter 12, but emphasis is on increasing physical activity and managing caloric intake.

   a.   Focus should be on consistent frequency of physical activity and choosing to do what can be enjoyed. Some examples of activities and calories used per minute of each activity are given in Table 10-1.

   b.   Although data remain sparse, a carbohydrate budget may be beneficial in the weight management of adolescents with PCOS. Whether this is due to specific carbohydrate effect alone or is associated with greater awareness of and consequent attention to total caloric decreased intake remains unclear.

D.   Diabetes mellitus develops much more frequently and at an earlier age in women with PCOS. Total cholesterol levels tend to be higher and HDL-cholesterol typically lower. Hypertension is three times more likely to develop. Clotting factor abnormalities resemble

Table 10-1.   Activity associated with calories used per minute of activity

Light activity (cal)	Medium activity (cal)	Strenuous activity (cal)
Dusting 2.5	Playing tennis 7.1	Cross-country run 10.6
Light housework 3.5	Gardening, digging 8.6	Cross-country ski 18.6
Slow dancing 5.2		
Golfing 5.0	Basketball 8.6	Walking up stairs 18.6

those seen in diabetes. Not surprisingly, heart disease is seen much more frequently in women with PCOS with estimates from a 4- to 11-fold increased risk. Weight contributes to the development of diabetes, high blood pressure, and cholesterol panel changes, so efforts at lifestyle management to decrease these risk factors are a priority in the treatment plan for PCOS.

II.   Reproductive years in the patient with diabetes mellitus revolve around the issue of either protecting against or preparing for conception and subsequent pregnancy management. Initial controversy as to safety of oral contraceptive use has led to studies showing that there is no reason that oral contraceptives should be specifically contraindicated in the woman with diabetes. Glycemic control may require adjustment of oral agent doses or adjustment of insulin, but for some women, the ability to stabilize hormonal fluctuations with oral contraceptive can actually result in more stable glycemic control. The luteal phase of the menstrual cycle has been associated with as much as a 30% increase in basal insulin dose in type 1 diabetes. This increased need, however, can precipitously drop within hours of menses onset, contributing to the erratic glucose pattern seen by women at different points in their cycle. Pregnancy should be planned with the goal of optimizing glycemic control before conception.

A.   Four percent of pregnant women had diabetes based on a national survey in the United States in 1988. Of these, 88% had gestational diabetes and 12% were prediagnosed diabetics with 35% having type 1 and 65% type 2. It is anticipated that as pregnancy is delayed into later years, fractionally even more women with type 2 diabetes will be seen. Early glycemic control is critical to prevent congenital anomalies and spontaneous abortion. As the pregnancy progresses, glycemic control is focused to prevent hypoglycemia and diabetic ketoacidosis. In the later stages of pregnancy, poor glycemic control has been associated with accelerated retinopathy, hypertension with increased pre-eclampsia/eclampsia, urinary tract infection including pyelonephritis, and polyhydramnios. At all stages, poor glycemic control is associated with increased risk of *in utero* fetal death.

B. **First-trimester** risks are those of unplanned pregnancy in the setting of suboptimal glucose control. Ideally, hemoglobin A1c (A1c) is targeted to <7.0% before conception. This is based on studies showing that if a glucose mean between 60 and 140 mg/dL could be attained, the incidence of anomalies was 1.2% if before conception versus 10.9% in women already pregnant who then attained these levels after conception. Neural tube defects specifically have occurred at the time of conception, although prevention of cardiac fetal abnormalities might be more amenable to immediate glucose normalization after conception.

    1. **Insulin** is the drug of choice. Oral agents have been reported to be safer than originally thought, but these studies need to be confirmed in larger series. Increasing insulin resistance during pregnancy will require insulin therapy at some point, so switching to insulin even before conception should be strongly considered in the patient not already using it. The starting dose should be 0.7 U/kg per day divided into three to four injections–preprandial short acting and bedtime longer acting. Glucose levels should be checked before and 1 hour after meals, at bedtime, and at 2 to 3 A.M. and dose adjustment made daily. Ideal goals of therapy are plasma glucose levels of 63 to 75 mg/dL before meal (capillary 55 to 65 mg/dL) and <140 mg/dL 1 hour after meal (capillary <120 mg/dL). Human insulin should be used. Reported results using insulin analogs are not yet available; however, as insulin pumps are increasingly being recommended for optimal glycemic control in pregnancy and the insulin used in these is typically either lispro or aspart, no differences to date have been evident in outcomes.

C. **As gestation progresses,** the insulin requirement will increase in a woman with type 1 diabetes to 0.8 U/kg per day through weeks 18 to 26, 0.9 U/kg per day through weeks 26 to 36, and 1.0 U/kg per day for the remaining weeks of pregnancy. Initial doses in significantly obese women may need to be much higher: 1.5 to 2.0 U/kg per day. In the type 2 diabetic, insulin needs will be similar in the first and second trimester and will be closer to 1.6 to 2.0 U/kg per day in the third trimester.

1.   A1c should be measured every 4 to 6 weeks and should decrease by 20% over the course of pregnancy, from the targeted initial 6.0% level.

2.   Dietary guidelines depend on preconception weight. If the woman is at ideal weight, daily intake should be 30 kcal/kg per day; if at 20% to 50% above ideal weight, then 24 kcal/kg per day; if over 50%, 12 to 18 kcal/kg per day. If the woman is >10% below ideal weight, then 36 to 40 kcal/kg per day is recommended. Although 40% to 50% of total calories should be carbohydrate, more often to control glucose, 40% appears to be more beneficial. Protein portion should be 20% and fat 30% to 40% of the remaining calories. Three meals and three snacks are the standard recommendation, with 10% total calories at breakfast, 30% at lunch, and 30% at dinner. Folate and iron supplementation should be encouraged.

3.   Exercise can be beneficial in decreasing insulin resistance, particularly in gestational diabetes. Although the benefit of exercise in a pregnant type 1 or 2 diabetic patient is not as clear, with potential for insulin-induced hypoglycemia, it may also mediate insulin resistance in the type 2 patient.

D.   Pregnancy-associated complications include retinopathy, hypertension, nephropathy, diabetic ketoacidosis, and thyroid dysfunction.

1.   Retinopathy in pregnancy has been associated with rapid normalization of glucose in the setting of increased insulin-like growth factor. In the Diabetes in Early Pregnancy Study, in 10.3% of women who progressed from a baseline of no retinopathy, initial A1c levels were 4 standard deviations above normal, and the longer the duration of diabetes history, the higher the risk of retinopathy progression. Additional identified risk factors include retinopathy at onset of pregnancy and proteinuria. Surveillance ophthalmology evaluation should be scheduled early in pregnancy and again in the second or third trimester as well as postpartum.

2.   Hypertension is defined as a blood pressure of greater than 120/80 mm Hg. If not treated, intrauterine growth retardation and fetal loss risk is increased. Medications used include hydralazine, methyldopa, β-blockers (particularly labetalol), and, after the first trimester, nifedipine. Angiotensin-converting inhibitors as well as angiotensin receptor blockers are contraindicated due to potential renal agenesis or renal failure in the fetus.

3.   Nephropathy, when not associated with hypertension, impacts fetal outcome only when clearance is <50 mL/min. Proteinuria of >250 mg per 24 hours in the first trimester has been associated with nephrotic syndrome in late pregnancy, requiring bedrest and at times parenteral protein replacement to prevent fetal hydrops.

4. **Diabetic ketoacidosis** is associated with high mortality risk for the fetus. Decreased intelligence has been linked to ketonemia during pregnancy. Women should be instructed to check routinely for ketones and to call promptly if moderate to large ketones are seen.

5. **Thyroid disease,** particularly subclinical hypothyroidism, occurs frequently in pregnant type 1 diabetic patients, with reported prevalence from 10% to 25%. Screening for hypothyroidism as well as hyperthyroidism should be done early in pregnancy with serum thyrotropin (thyroid-stimulating hormone), although this test might be falsely depressed in the first weeks following conception. Serial determinations are helpful in determining actual thyroid levels if the thyroid-stimulating hormone level is initially low.

E. **Fetal surveillance** through ultrasound can estimate age if done before the twenty-eighth week, screen for structural abnormalities, evaluate growth, assess amniotic fluid, and determine fetal status dynamically through Doppler and biophysical studies. Two percent of diabetic pregnancies (in contrast to 0.1% to 0.2% of nondiabetic pregnancies) will have neural tube defects. Other increased congenital anomalies in diabetic pregnancies are anencephaly, microencephaly, caudal regression syndrome, and genitourinary and gastrointestinal anomalies. Hypertrophic cardiomyopathy, atrial and ventricular septal defects, transposition of the great vessels, and coarctation of the aorta are the more typical diabetic pregnancy-associated congenital heart diseases. Hydramnios is associated with fetal hyperglycemia. When to start antepartum surveillance varies according to physician and clinical status. If glycemic control has been poor, testing is often started as early as 26 to 28 weeks; in the woman with excellent control, testing is often deferred to the thirty-fifth week.

F. During **labor and delivery,** glucose control is important to minimize neonatal hypoglycemia. Insulin is often given by infusion with the goal of maintaining glucose level between 70 and 90 mg/dL. Often a rate of only 1 to 3 U per hour is needed, and as labor progresses, this may be discontinued and glucose may have to be given to prevent maternal hypoglycemia resulting from rapidly decreasing insulin resistance from placental expulsion, to maintain goal glucose concentration.

G. Postpartum, it is not unusual to see normo-glycemia for 24 to 72 hours despite no insulin even in type 1 diabetic patients. Resumption of insulin at 0.6 U/kg of postpartum weight per day can be accompanied by caloric recommendation of 25 kcal/kg per day (27 kcal/kg per day if breastfeeding).

III.   Menopause in diabetic women occurs at the same time as in women without diabetes. Observational data supporting the benefit of estrogen replacement in women with diabetes are potentially fraught with the same problem as in nondiabetic women, in whom randomized, controlled trials of both the Women's Health Initiative and the Heart and Estrogen Replacement Study not only did not support hormonal replacement as adding benefit clinically but raised serious issues as to the safety of postmenopausal hormone therapy. In a subset of women enrolled in the Study of Osteoporotic Fractures, who had diabetes and were 65 years of age and older, follow-up over 12 years showed that the women with diabetes had a 42% increased risk of incident disability. They were more likely than women without diabetes to report being unable to perform tasks such as walking or climbing stairs or even cooking meals. Although obesity, coronary heart disease, physical inactivity, arthritis, and severe visual impairment were each independently associated with disability, having diabetes mellitus at an age not currently being temporally categorized as frail elderly seemed more likely to place the postmenopausal woman into this category. However, physical interventions including balance and strength training have improved physical function in elderly diabetic patients. This needs further investigation as older women with diabetes are more likely to fall, with some studies, although not all, suggesting greater potential for injury from falls in this population.

Cognitive function has been shown to diminish more in women with uncontrolled hyperglycemia than in women with lower A1c values. Long-term memory loss has been shown to affect more elderly women with impaired glucose tolerance than women with normal glucose tolerance. Urinary tract infections occur more frequently in postmenopausal women with diabetes than without diabetes. This is irrespective of duration of diabetes, but increased frequency was seen in women who were treated with oral glycemic control agents or insulin, not in those managing their diabetes through lifestyle. Women with diabetes have a shortened lifespan, but it is not clear whether this is due to the diabetes itself or the co-morbidities of vascular disease. Further work is needed to clarify these issues.

SELECTED READING

American Diabetes Association. Preconception care of women with diabetes. *Diabetes Care* 2002;25(suppl 1):S82–S84.

Boyko EJ, Fihn SD, Scholles D, et al. Diabetes and the risk of acute urinary tract infection among postmenopausal women. *Diabetes Care* 2002;25:1778–1783.

Dunaif A, Thomas A. Current concepts in the polycystic ovarian syndrome. *Annu Rev Med* 2001;52:401–419.

Franks S. Polycystic ovarian syndrome. *N Engl J Med* 1995;333: 853–861.

Gregg EW, Mangione CM, Cauley JA, et al. Diabetes and incidence of functional disability in older women. *Diabetes Care* 2002;25:61–67.

Jovanovic L. Medical emergencies in the patient with diabetes during pregnancy. *Endocrinol Metab Clin North Am* 2000;29: 771–785.

Legro RS. Polycystic ovarian syndrome. Phenotype to genotype. *Endocrinol Clin North Am* 1999;28:379–396.

Schwartz AV, Hillier TA, Sellmeyer DE, et al. Older women and diabetes have a higher risk of falls: a prospective study. *Diabetes Care* 2002;25:1749–1754.

Men and Diabetes

I. Puberty. Type 1 diabetes affects both genders equally. It can occur at any age, but it has its peak incidence in late childhood/early adolescence, with the peak being somewhat earlier in girls than in boys. After initiation of insulin therapy, normal growth and sexual development depend more on the presence of adequate insulinization than on the achievement of near-normal glycemia. Early reports suggested that children with type 1 diabetes grew more slowly than their nondiabetic peers, entered puberty at a later age, and achieved a significantly decreased final adult height. The most severe example of this is the Mauriac syndrome, consisting of hepatomegaly, growth failure, and pubertal delay. This syndrome is now quite rare and is related to profound underinsulinization. Most children currently display normal growth patterns with normal onset and progression of pubertal development. In the Diabetes Control and Complications Trial, the adolescent boys receiving intensive therapy with multiple injections or insulin pump therapy gained 4.04 kg more than their conventionally treated peers (who received one or two daily injections). It is also interesting to note that studies comparing adolescent boys and girls almost universally find lower hemoglobin A1c levels for the boys.

II. Young adulthood. This is a time when one searches for a place in society. Finding a mate, establishing a family, and initiating a career are major tasks to be accomplished. Young men with diabetes who abuse drugs or alcohol pose significant challenges to their health care providers. Alcohol-related accidents among young adults (with and without diabetes) continue to be the leading cause of death in this age group. Motor vehicle accidents in the late teen years and early twenties are much more common in males than females. A young man with diabetes is therefore potentially more dangerous drinking, driving, and potentially hypoglycemic. It is therefore critical to discuss this situation with the young man and the need for frequent blood glucose testing both prior to driving and while drinking alcohol. A discussion of how alcohol may affect blood glucose (inhibition of hepatic gluconeogenesis resulting in a greater risk for hypoglycemia) should be considered for almost all adolescents and young adults.

III.   Male reproduction. There are no data to suggest that men with diabetes have more infertility than men without diabetes. Erectile dysfunction (ED), however, is much more common in older men with diabetes.

   A.   Erectile dysfunction
      1.   Prevalence. The frequency of ED in diabetes was evaluated in a survey of 541 diabetic men aged 20 to 59 years attending a large community diabetes clinic. The prevalence of ED increased progressively with age, from 6% in men aged 20 to 24 years to 52% in men aged 55 to 59 years. In addition to increasing age, the main factors associated with ED were peripheral or autonomic neuropathy, retinopathy, long duration of diabetes, and poor glycemic control. A larger more recent study reported that for men over the age of 50 years, increasing duration of diabetes was the greatest risk for ED.
      2.   Etiology. ED can result from local nerve damage (neuropathy or surgical trauma), impaired blood flow to the penis, or psychological factors; several of these factors are present in most cases.
      3.   Evaluation. Many men with ED go undiagnosed due to embarrassment about discussing sexual function. It is appropriate to discuss this topic with all men with diabetes. Furthermore, if present, the physician should not assume the ED is caused by diabetes. A proper history assesses other potential etiologies, several of which are reversible. Any possible etiology for hypogonadism should be entertained. An appropriate history would include questions about libido and headaches. Furthermore, a complete history of drug use and alcohol consumption should be discussed. The history should also include symptoms of vascular disease (especially claudication) and neuropathy. Although an expensive laboratory evaluation is often recommended, the most important testing would include serum testosterone, prolactin, and thyrotropin levels. Different series in the literature report anywhere from 4% to 29% of men with ED having some type of hormonal abnormality responsible for the ED. Symptoms of hypogonadism do not differentiate those with or without low levels of testosterone, so hormonal testing should be done on all men with a complaint of ED.

4.   Treatments

a.   Hormonal. Hypogonadism is not more common in men with diabetes. However, obese men with diabetes are common, and obesity leads to an abnormal binding with sex hormone-binding globulin. For this reason, obese men should have serum free testosterone rather than total testosterone levels measured. If the serum free testosterone level is low, treating it with intramuscular or topical testosterone will often be effective. However, it is perhaps more important to determine the etiology of the hypogonadism. A complete discussion of this topic is beyond the scope of this chapter, but at the very least, one should differentiate primary from secondary hypogonadism with the measurement of gonadotropins and prolactin, thyroid function studies, and possibly imaging of the pituitary gland.

b.   Sildenafil (Viagra). This drug is a cyclic GMP phosphodiesterase inhibitor that prolongs the vasodilatory effect of nitric oxide to initiate and maintain an erection. Overall, results of efficacy in men with diabetes are slightly less than in their nondiabetic counterparts. For example, in one large study with 268 men with diabetes, sildenafil was effective at improving erections in 56% of subjects compared with 10% of subjects assigned placebo. For most patients, the recommended dose is 50 mg taken as needed, approximately 1 hour before sexual activity. However, sildenafil may be taken anywhere from 30 minutes to 4 hours before sexual activity. Based on effectiveness and tolerance, the dose may be increased to a maximum recommended dose of 100 mg or decreased to 25 mg. The maximum recommended dosing frequency is once daily. Because of its high efficacy rate and relative safety, the expensive vascular and neurologic workups from 20 years ago are now obsolete.

(1)   **Adverse effects.** Most side effects are related to the vasodilatory effects of the drug. The most common adverse events are headache, lightheadedness, dizziness, flushing, and, in some cases, syncope. Men at highest risk for syncope are those who take other vasodilators such as nitrates. With the 100-mg dose, there are also complaints of distorted vision.

c.   Intraurethral alprostadil (Caverject, Edex, Muse pellet). Also indicated for the treatment of ED, there are no diabetes-specific data published for this agent. Major side effects include flushing and penile pain, although bradycardia, dizziness, and headaches are also reported.

d. Intracavernosal injections. There are several approved agents for the treatment of ED with intracavernosal injections. These treatments include papaverine, phentolamine, and alprostadil. However, with the availability of sildenafil and more GMP phosphodiesterase inhibitors under development, these agents are used infrequently now.

SELECTED READING

Bacon CG, Hu BG, Giovannucci E, et al. Association of type and duration of diabetes with erectile dysfunction in a large cohort of men. *Diabetes Care* 2002;25:1458–1463.

Carbone DJ, Seftel AD. Erectile dysfunction. Diagnosis and treatment in older men. *Geriatrics* 2002;57:18–24.

Rendell MS, Rajfer J, Wicker PA, et al. Sildenafil for treatment of erectile dysfunction in men with diabetes: a randomized controlled trial. Sildenafil Diabetes Study Group. *JAMA* 1999;281:421–426.

Prevention of Diabetes

Increasing evidence is accumulating that diabetes mellitus can be prevented or at least delayed through a number of interventions. Type 2 diabetes can be prevented or delayed through lifestyle management, medication intervention, even the avoidance of specific behaviors. Prevention of type 1 diabetes has also been shown in various observational studies, although specific intervention with low-dose insulin was disappointing in the Diabetes Prevention Trial 1.

    I. Lifestyle modification as related specifically to weight loss and increase in physical activity has been shown in three separate randomized trials. The Diabetes Prevention Pilot Study centered in the United States showed a 58% reduction in progression from impaired glucose tolerance to diabetes with targets of 7% weight loss and 150 minutes of exercise per week over a 3-year period. In a Finnish cohort, an intervention aimed at weight reduction of ≥5%, intake of total fat of <30% and saturated fat of <10% of total calories ingested, increase in fiber to ≥15 g/1,000 kcal, and exercise for at least 30 minutes per day also resulted in a similar 58% reduction in the progression from impaired glucose tolerance to diabetes mellitus over 4 years. In the Da Qing Impaired Glucose Tolerance and Diabetes Study, in which randomization was by clinic rather than by individual, over 6 years, there was a 46% decrease in progression to diabetes with interventions of diet, exercise, or diet and exercise. Unanswered questions are whether these interventions are sustainable over time as well as whether they remain as effective. However, the similarity in the numbers of individuals of various ethnicities, genders, and risk factors in whom diabetes was prevented or at best delayed is striking.

    A. This information has been taken by the public as an impetus for behavior change benefit even in at-risk situations of development of autoimmune type 1 diabetes, where scientific evidence would support no such lifestyle benefit. Among 400 first-degree relatives of type 1 diabetic individuals invited to participate in measurement of their immune markers, when questioned how they might use their information as to being at high risk for type 1, 87% responded with planned changes related to diet (i.e., eating and drinking habits, decreased sugar consumption) and 30% responded with planned lifestyle change (increased exercise level), suggesting strong belief in the benefit of lifestyle change as protective against diabetes, although data support benefit only for type 2.

II. Medications used in the treatment of diabetes and associated co-morbidities have also shown preventative benefits.

A. Among oral glycemic control agents, metformin, acarbose, and troglitazone have been shown to decrease progression from impaired glucose tolerance to diabetes mellitus. In the Diabetes Prevention Pilot Study, metformin decreased progression to diabetes by 31%. In obese adolescents with insulin resistance and positive history of diabetes in first- or second-degree family members, use of metformin was associated with weight loss and lower fasting glucose levels, although insulin resistance remained unchanged during the time of study. Acarbose has also been shown to reduce progression from impaired glucose tolerance to diabetes during a 3-year follow-up in the Study to Prevent Non-Insulin-Dependent Diabetes Mellitus. However, after a 3-month subsequent washout period in which acarbose was discontinued in the treatment group, the rate of conversion to diabetes was higher in the previously treated group than in the nontreated group, suggesting that acarbose might have masked diabetes rather than prevented it. In the Troglitazone in Prevention of Diabetes (TRIPOD) Study, interruption of troglitazone for 8 months was still associated with less progression to diabetes among women with previous gestational diabetes.

B. In the Heart Outcomes Prevention Evaluation (HOPE) trial, a retrospective study of 5,720 individuals randomized to **ramipril** or placebo showed that only 3.6% developed diabetes on ramipril as compared with 5.4% on placebo ($p < 0.001$). In individuals with known diabetes at trial entry, hemoglobin A1c values were 0.2%. Statins might also be protective, as participants in the West of Scotland Coronary Prevention Study using **pravastatin** had a 30% decrease in the development of diabetes. However, both of these findings were from *post hoc* analyses, and prospective trials are required for confirmation. Given that both statins and angiotensin-converting enzyme inhibitors have anti-inflammatory effects, this might explain the diabetes-protective effect. In the Women's Health

Study, those in the highest quartile for C-reactive protein and interleukin-6, both markers of inflammation, had relative risks of 15.7% and 7.5%, respectively, of progressing to diabetes, even after adjustment for family history of diabetes, exercise, body mass index, alcohol use, and hormone replacement therapy.

C.   Associated with decreased risk of development of type 1 diabetes is observational data that **cod liver oil** used during pregnancy decreases development of type 1 in offspring by 60% up to 15 years of age. Two thousand international units of vitamin D supplementation in a northern Finnish cohort study was associated with an 80% reduction in development of diabetes in infants followed from birth to 1 year of age. Vitamin D is known to have immunologic properties, although potential toxicity warrants care in its use.

D.   Intriguing data, although of short-term observation, involve **heat shock protein therapy** in the early diagnosis of type 1 diabetes and associated preservation of β-cell function.

III.   Specific behaviors   have been associated with development of diabetes, mostly from long-term observational data. The Nurses Health Study, involving 85,000 women followed over 16 years, showed that smoking, a body mass index over 25,   and exercising a half-hour or less per week were all correlated with higher risk for the development of diabetes. Protective factors included moderate alcohol intake, increased cereal fiber intake, decreased trans-fatty food intake, and use of foods with increased polyunsaturated-to-saturated fatty acid content. Nut and peanut butter consumption has specifically been pointed out as protective, although these same women were typically thinner and ingested more fiber, more magnesium, alcohol, and fewer trans-fatty foods. They also ate less meat and refined grain products. Among men in the Health Professionals Follow-Up Study followed over 12 years, a diet high in red meat, processed meat, high-fat dairy products, french fries, refined grains, and sweets and desserts was associated with a 20% to 60% increased risk of diabetes, increasing with each quintile of higher intake. However, increased dairy consumption in overweight young adults has been associated inversely with the risk of type 2 diabetes, suggesting limits to observational data.

SELECTED READING

Chiasson J-L, Josse RG, Gomis R, et al. Acarbose for prevention of type 2 diabetes mellitus: the STOP-NIDDM randomized trial. *Lancet* 2002;359:2072–2077.

Hypponen E, Laara E, Reunanen A, et al. Intake of vitamin D and risk of type 1 diabetes: a birth cohort study. *Lancet* 2001;358: 1500–1503.

Knowler WC, Barrett–Connor E, Fowler SE, et al. The Diabetes Prevention Program Research Group. Reduction in the incidence of type 2 diabetes with lifestyle intervention or metformin. *N Engl J Med* 2002;346:393–403.

Pan XR, Li G-W, Hu Y-H, et al. The Da Qing IGT and Diabetes Study: effects of diet and exercise in preventing NIDDM in people with impaired glucose tolerance. *Diabetes Care* 1997;20: 537–544.

Pereira MA, Jacobs DR, Van Horn L, et al. Dairy consumption, obesity, and the insulin resistance syndrome in young adults. The CARDIA Study. *JAMA* 2002;287:2081–2089.

Tuomilehto J, Lindstrom J, Eriksson JG, et al. Prevention of diabetes mellitus by changes in lifestyle among subjects with impaired glucose tolerance. *N Engl J Med* 2001;344:1343–1350.

van Dam RM, Rimm EB, Willett WC, et al. Dietary patterns and risk for type 2 diabetes mellitus in U.S. men. *Ann Intern Med* 2002;136:201–209.

Yusuf S, Gerstein H, Hoogwerf B, et al. Ramipril and the development of diabetes. *JAMA* 2001;286:1882–1885.

The Future of Diabetes Care

I.   **New medications for the treatment of hyper-glycemia**

   A.   **Oral agents.** Novel insulin sensitizers are now being developed. Drugs that do not cause weight gain (in a population already obese) but improve both resistance to insulin and the atherogenic lipid profile would be ideal. At the current time, we are seeing a plethora of combination agents, but these do not really add anything to our pharmacologic armamentarium. Included in this category would have to be the possibility of oral insulin, an idea that has been elusive for over 80 years but that is being actively pursued.

   B.   **Parenteral medications.** We will see a variety of new insulin analogs over the next few years, which, like our initial analogs, should improve insulin therapy and give both patients and their providers more choices to reach glycemic targets without excessive hypoglycemia. Besides new insulins, there will be several "insulin enhancers," which will be administered subcutaneously and have beneficial effects on glycemia. An analog to the hormone amylin seems to improve blood glucose, as do analogs to the hormone glucagon-like peptide-1. Initial data with the latter peptide show great promise for patients with type 2 diabetes in particular, as besides improving glycemia, there tend to be decreases in weight. Furthermore, initial data with these latter agents suggest they are truly β-cell sparing. Besides analogs to glucagon-like peptide-1, there is also interest in pharmacologic agents that act by inhibiting the enzyme that degrades this peptide.

   C.   **Inhaled medications.** One of the most elusive goals has been the introduction of inhaled insulin. Several companies are now trying to perfect this technology. One of the problems has been that relatively small amounts of insulin are able to penetrate the lung tissue; thus, large doses of insulin must be inhaled through an inhaler. Pulmonary function and insulin antibody levels have been other concerns. There is also a company studying the possibility of buccal insulin delivery, which is not technically inhaled. Oral insulin is yet another possibility, now being actively pursued.

II.   New technologies for the treatment of hyperglycemia

   A.   Glucose sensors. There is increasing excitement about the use of glucose sensors to help improve diabetes control. This technology is still in its infancy. Although two types of sensors are currently available, their use is limited. It is expected this technology will improve over time while costs decrease, allowing more "real-time" glucose data that are accurate and able to better predict insulin requirements due to the ability to trend the "glycemic slope."

   B.   Implantable pumps. This technology has been slow to develop due to problems with insulin occlusion after implantation. However, improvements in the insulin make this technology much more feasible. The goal is to have an implantable pump that communicates with a glucose sensor, thus creating an "artificial pancreas." This concept has been discussed for years; trials are now underway in Europe.

III.   New technologies for home blood glucose monitoring data management

   A.   Computerized downloads. Although available for many years, this is one technology that has been underutilized. As patients learn the importance of increasing the frequency of their home blood glucose monitoring, downloaded meter data allow visualization of data not apparent from a written logbook. At the current time, all of the meter companies have software that allows providers to download their patients' meters, but more patients are using the software for this themselves for assistance in their diabetes control. With the increased use of personalized digital assistants (PDAs), many companies are now allowing communication of meter data with the PDA. The PDA in turn can also be used to store other data not routinely found on the meter, including the carbohydrate content of many foods, even items from popular restaurants. Finally, data from insulin pumps (insulin rates, insulin boluses) will also be able to communicate with PDAs.

   B.   "Smart" insulin pens. Insulin pens have been available in the United States since the mid-1980s, but only after the turn of the century have they been used with any frequency. This is in contrast to Europe, where pen usage is much more common. Pens that can track insulin doses, both to allow patients to recall how much insulin was taken at what time and for downloads into computers, will be available in the future. Furthermore, matching the data from the pen with a glucose meter should also be possible.

IV.   New medications for the treatment of complications

   A.   Protein kinase C inhibitors. Until now, using specific medications to treat microvascular complications, macrovascular disease, or neuropathy has not been successful. Studies to date using advanced glycation product inhibitors and aldose reductase blockers have shown minimal benefit with many adverse events. Currently, studies are underway using a different strategy, protein kinase C inhibition, to determine if these agents can slow or possibly reverse a variety of different diabetes-related complications.

   V.   Islet cell transplants. Certainly, the possibility of islet cell transplants to cure type 1 diabetes has been a goal for many decades. The success of the group in Edmonton, Canada, has provided hope to many families. Much work still needs to be completed, however, before this can be a realistic option for large populations of patients. Concerns about immunosuppression and the availability of sufficient islets are the main obstacles. Still, there has been much recent progress, and the realization of this therapy as an option for patients with type 1 diabetes remains an important research objective.

SELECTED READING

Baron AD, Kim D, Weyer C. Novel peptides under development for the treatment of type 1 and type 2 diabetes. *Curr Drug Targets Immune Endocr Metab Disord* 2002;2:63–82.

Cefalu WT, Skyler JS, Kourides IA, et al. Inhaled human insulin treatment in patients with type 2 diabetes mellitus. *Ann Intern Med* 2001;134:203–207.

Kim SK. Pancreatic islet cell replacement: successes and opportunities. *Ann NY Acad Sci* 2002;961:41–43.

Klonoff DC. Current, emerging, and future trends in metabolic monitoring. *Diabetes Technol Ther* 2002;4:583–588.

Robert JJ. Continuous monitoring of blood glucose. *Horm Res* 2002;57(suppl 1):81–84.

Appendix

Diabetes and You: Basic Information for Patients Coping with Diabetes

Diagnosis and Maintenance

What Are the Main Types of Diabetes?

There are several different types of diabetes, and different terms are used to describe each of them. Here are some of the most common ones.

Type 1, or insulin-dependent diabetes. This is most common in children and young adults, but can occur at any age. It occurs because the insulin-producing cells in the pancreas are destroyed by the person's own immune system, eventually resulting in a complete loss of insulin secretion. People with type 1 diabetes have to take insulin shots at least once a day to stay healthy and keep the blood glucose levels near normal. Their life is truly dependent on insulin.

Type 2, or non-insulin–dependent diabetes. This is the most common of all forms of diabetes. It usually occurs in middle-aged or elderly adults, especially those who are overweight. We are not sure exactly what causes type 2 diabetes. People with it do make some insulin, but make less than they need. In addition, many of their body tissues become resistant to the effects of insulin. For these reasons, many people with this non-insulin—dependent diabetes do require insulin treatment. Sometimes type 2 people require supplemental insulin as a part of their diabetes treatment. They are called "insulin requiring."

"Secondary" diabetes. Diabetes can occur if people have another disease of their pancreas. Diseases such as cystic fibrosis, pancreatitis (inflammation of the pancreas), and pancreatic cancer may destroy enough of the insulin-producing cells to cause diabetes. An excess of steroid hormones in the blood can occur if someone is taking steroid drugs (like prednisone) or if someone has a steroid-producing tumor. In these situations, the excess steroids prevent insulin from working properly and so cause diabetes.

Gestational diabetes. Some women develop diabetes during pregnancy. It is important that this is diagnosed and treated to ensure a good outcome and a healthy baby. Although the diabetes goes away after delivery, women who have gestational diabetes are at increased risk of developing type 2 diabetes in later life.

Impaired glucose tolerance. This is a condition in which the fasting blood glucose level is slightly above normal, or between 110 and 126 mg/dL. About 25% of the persons with impaired glucose tolerance later develop diabetes.

Diabetes Treatment Targets

	Nondiabetic	ADA[a]
HbA1c	4%–6%	Below 7%
Before-meal glucose	Below 110 mg/dL	90–130 mg/dL
Bedtime glucose	Below 120 mg/dL	110–180 mg/dL
LDL-cholesterol	Below 100 mg/dL	Below 100 mg/dL
HDL-cholesterol (men)	Above 40 mg/dL	Above 40 mg/dL
HDL-cholesterol (women)	Above 50 mg/dL	Above 50 mg/dL
Triglycerides	Below 150 mg/dL	Below 150 mg/dL
Blood pressure	Below 130/80	Below 130/80
Foot check		Yearly
Urine protein screen		Yearly
Dilated eye exam		At diagnosis, then yearly[b]

[a]American Diabetes Association treatment targets in 2003.
[b]For type 1 diabetes, initial examination within 3 to 5 years of diagnosis once over age 10 years, then yearly.

YOUR CURRENT TARGETS

HbA1c:
Before-meal glucose:
Bedtime glucose:
LDL cholesterol:
HDL-cholesterol (men):
HDL-cholesterol (women):
Triglycerides:
Blood pressure:
Foot check:
Urine protein screening:
Dilated eye exam:

Reasons for Testing Blood Glucose Levels

There are many reasons for monitoring your blood glucose levels. Some of the reasons include the following:

1. It helps you be involved in your diabetes management. It helps you learn how food, activity, medicines, stress, and illness affect diabetes control.
2. It helps to tailor your target blood glucose goals.
3. It can be used for both type 1 and type 2 diabetes and with all types of therapy.
4. It can help to prevent acute complications such as ketoacidosis and hypoglycemia.
5. It helps to prevent or detect hypoglycemia in those with "hypoglycemia unawareness."
6. It is *much* more accurate than urine glucose *testing*.
7. This type of monitoring is vital during pregnancy and with insulin pumps.
8. You will know the results right away.
9. The results are accurate if the test is done correctly and the meter is working properly.
10. It is very useful in identifying low and high blood glucose patterns.

HOME BLOOD GLUCOSE TESTING

One of the most exciting developments in diabetes management is home blood glucose (sugar) testing. At one time, urine glucose testing was widely used by patients to provide guidance in the adjustment of medication dosage. Since then, diabetes specialists have found urine testing far too inaccurate to rely on because many factors can falsely elevate or lower urine test results. Home blood glucose testing has been available for many years and is highly accurate. All people with diabetes can benefit immensely by learning this simple technique. We will work with you to select the most appropriate testing equipment (meter, test strip, lancet, and finger-stick device).

The seconds to 1- to 2-minute procedure involves an almost painless finger stick, placement of a droplet of blood onto a test strip, and a visual or electronic meter readout of the result. You will then record your result in a diary or logbook. In this way, we learn together how food activity, medication, stress, and other factors affect your blood.

Some of the features to consider when choosing a meter are the following:

- Memory
- Cost
- Size
- Speed
- Accuracy

There are different technologies in meters. Your health care provider may suggest one that will best meet your needs.

When Caring for Your Meter and Test Strips, Be Sure to:

1. Clean and calibrate the machine each week. If more frequent testing occurs, increase the number of cleaning and care times.
2. Have a spare set of batteries on hand.
3. Avoid exposing meter or strips to extremes in temperature or humidity. Keep them away from direct sun. Do not leave them in a hot car. Extreme cold in winter can affect or alter readings. Let your meter warm up first.
4. Keep strips sealed in their original container when not in use.
5. Carry your meter and strips in the protective case that comes with your meter.

To Clean Your Meter:

1. Use a damp cloth and then dry well.
2. Do not use alcohol to clean the meter.
3. Change test strip holder if needed.
4. Do not take the meter apart to fix it.

The proper maintenance of the meter ensures more accurate readings. Each meter should come with directions. If you need help, ask your health care provider.

HOME URINE KETONE TESTING

People with type 1 (insulin-dependent) diabetes also learn how to test their own urine sample for ketones (acetone). Normally, the body uses glucose (sugar) as its main source of energy or fuel. For the glucose to be used, sufficient insulin must be present to allow the glucose to enter body cells. If there is a lack or a deficiency of insulin, the body will begin to burn stored fat instead of glucose as its energy source.

Ketones result from the breakdown of fat and are not normally present in blood or urine. The presence of ketones in the urine indicates the breakdown of fat, usually due to a lack of insulin. This can result from problems such as onset of type 1 diabetes, illness, incorrect dosage or administration of insulin, or fasting.

The presence of urine ketones is a serious sign. It may indicate that a life-threatening condition is developing and should be reported to your health care provider promptly. There are test strips that patients can dip into a small urine sample, which will indicate if ketones are present; the procedure takes only 15 seconds.

1. Dip a test strip into a fresh sample of urine.
2. Wait the number of seconds indicated in the instructions. If there are ketones in your urine, the color of the pad on the test strip will change.
3. Compare the color on the pad with the color chart of the bottle or box.
4. Record the test result in your logbook.

If you find ketones in your urine, it is a sign that you need to improve your blood glucose control. If large or moderate ketones are present, call your health care provider right away. If you are able to drink, push sugar-free fluids. Also see Basic Sick Day Rules for guidelines.

Test Your Urine for Ketones When:

- Your blood glucose is over 240 mg/dL.
- You are sick.
- You are pregnant.
- If told to do so by your provider.

How to Dispose of Syringes, Needles, and Lancets

Accidental or deliberate skin puncture with used needles or lancets can cause the spread of very serious diseases such as hepatitis and AIDS. This can happen whether the puncture is accidental or deliberate.

Your insulin syringes, needles, and lancets should never be thrown away in your regular trash or waste containers because these could cause accidental needle sticks in the people who collect the containers. Even if you clip off your needles with a special device, a small sharp "nub" may remain and be a hazard. You could be fined or otherwise penalized for improper disposal of "sharps," or your trash may not be picked up. Follow these guidelines for proper and safe disposal of your used supplies:

- Never share your supplies with anyone else. If you use needles or lancets that were already used by someone else, you risk developing serious diseases such as hepatitis and AIDS, which are spread by direct contact with infected blood.
- All needles and other sharps can be collected and stored in a coffee can, plastic soda pop bottle, empty bleach bottle, or special sharps container. Containers must have the lid in place, be labeled, and be sealed with duct or similar tape.
- Ask your health care team where you can safely dispose of your sharps container. Different rules and regulations exist for every community.

The "Three-Month Blood Sugar Test"

HEMOGLOBIN A1C

The hemoglobin A1c (A1c or HbA1c) test gives your doctor, care team, and you an accurate measure of your overall diabetes control. This test measures the amount of glucose that is attached to the red blood cells. These cells live in the bloodstream for about 120 days. Glucose that is not used for energy and is left in the blood attaches itself to proteins that are part of the cells. When glucose levels have been high, more and more red blood cells have glucose attached to them. As a result, the A1c level gives an estimate of blood glucose levels for the last 2 to 3 months. Unlike your regular blood sugar tests, the A1c is not affected by short-term changes such as a meal you ate right before the test.

"Normal range" in the A1c test means the expected test result in a person without diabetes. This range can vary from laboratory to laboratory. Be sure to ask what the "normal range" is at the laboratory your doctor uses.

You should have this test done every 3 to 6 months. Ask your doctor how often you should have it done. Also ask what your result was the last time your A1c was measured.

The A1c result can show if you are doing a good overall job of managing your diabetes. Sometimes it also helps detect meter problems or accuracy problems in daily home blood glucose tests.

Low Blood Sugar (Hypoglycemia) and Type 2 Diabetes

Sometimes your blood sugar can get too low. Low blood sugar may cause you to feel shaky, weak or sweaty and/or have blurred vision. You may also feel anxious, cranky, light-headed, confused, angry, and/or numb around the mouth. You may feel many or only one of these signs. Low blood sugar can happen when you have skipped or are late with a meal or snack or when you have done extra work or exercise.

If this happens to you, check your blood sugar level. If it is > 80 mg/dL, your blood sugar is not low. Your body is reacting to a blood sugar that is lower than normal for you. If you sit down and relax, the uncomfortable feelings go away.

If your blood sugar is < 80 mg/dL, eat or drink a small amount of food with carbohydrates. Some choices are listed.

Food	Amount
Glucose tablets	3 tabs
Insta Glucose Gel	½ tube
Honey	1 tbsp
Fruit juice	½ cup
Soft drink, regular	¾ cup

Carry one of these foods with you at all times. Low blood sugar comes on very quickly. If this happens more than one hour before a meal, also eat half a sandwich or drink 1 cup of nonfat milk.

High-fat and -calorie foods (such as ice cream, candy, Snickers, M&Ms, sweet desserts, etc.) are not good to treat low blood sugar. The fat in these foods slows the absorption of sugar and slows the rise in blood sugar. The extra calories can increase your weight. Also, you may be tempted to eat those foods in excess, which can cause your blood sugar to rise to high levels.

Low Blood Sugar (Hypoglycemia) and Type 1 Diabetes

SYMPTOMS

The symptoms of hypoglycemia vary, and they may even vary for the same person over time. Common symptoms include the following:

- Shaking
- Sweating
- Nausea
- Hunger
- Heart pounding

Other symptoms that usually (but not always) occur later include the following:

- Blurred vision
- Confusion
- Tiredness
- Anxiety

Some patients lose the ability to recognize these symptoms, and this is called "hypoglycemia unawareness." We know that some patients who have had diabetes for >10 years do not recognize their hypoglycemia because of neuropathy (damage to the nerve fibers). We are now beginning to appreciate that hypoglycemia unawareness is common in many more individuals than previously thought. It is especially common in individuals who try to keep their blood glucose levels in near-normal ranges. The reason for this is *not yet* entirely clear. Therefore, should you and your physician decide you want to achieve "tight" blood glucose control, it will be important for you to measure your blood glucose levels frequently each day. This will minimize your risk for hypoglycemia.

If you do not feel right, or if you are just "feeling funny," it is important to measure your blood sugar. Your "funny feeling" might be caused by a dropping blood glucose level. If a blood glucose meter is not available, the best strategy is to treat yourself as if you were having a hypoglycemia episode.

How to Treat Your Hypoglycemia

Hypoglycemia is treated by eating foods with carbohydrates. Fifteen grams of concentrated carbohydrate will raise your blood glucose to a reasonable level in 10 to 30 minutes. Foods that provide 15 g of carbohydrate are listed below. Foods high in glucose (i.e., glucose tablets, Insta Glucose Gel, honey) have the quickest effect on low blood sugar. A meal or snack should be eaten 30 to 60 minutes following treatment of hypoglycemia.

Carbohydrate source	Amount	Glucose (g)	Carbo-hydrate	Calories
Glucose tablets	3 tabs	15.0	15.0	60
Insta Glucose (Gel)	½ - to 31-g tube	6.4	12.5	50
Gelatin, regular, prepared	½ cup	6.0	17.0	71
Honey	1 tbsp	7.1	17.3	64
Juice				
Apple	½ cup	3.1	14.5	58
Orange	½ cup	6.6	12.8	54
Milk, skim	1 cup	0	12.0	85
Raisins	2 tbsp	5.6	14.2	54
Soft drinks, regular				
Cola	½ cup	5.0	12.8	50
Ginger ale	¾ cup	7.4	15.9	52
Sugar, brown, packed	1 tbsp	0.7	13.2	51
Syrup, corn	1 tbsp	4.1	15.0	44
Thirst quencher	1 cup	5.8	15.2	60

Low Blood Sugar (Hypoglycemia) in the Middle of the Night

Hypoglycemia in the middle of the night is first treated with 15 g of carbohydrate—the same as during the day. You also need an extra 15 g of carbohydrate and 10 g of protein. This extra food should prevent further hypoglycemia during the night. The table below gives some ideas for treating middle-of-the-night hypoglycemia.

Carbohydrate source	Amount	Carbohydrate	Calories
Glucose tablets	3 tabs		
and nonfat milk	1 cup	27	150
Honey,	1 tbsp		
crackers, and	4 each		
cheese	1 oz	32	294
Orange juice,	½ cup		
bread, and	1 slice		
ham	1 oz	30	210

Skipping, delaying, or reducing the size of meals and snacks is the most common cause of hypoglycemia. If a meal or snack is going to be late, eat something to avoid hypoglycemia.

Increased physical activity will lower blood glucose. The effect of exercise can lower blood glucose up to 36 hours after the activity.

Drinking alcohol, especially on an empty stomach, can cause hypoglycemia. Its effect on blood glucose can occur 3 to 8 hours after drinking. If you drink, be sure also to eat and drink only in moderation.

What You Need to Know About High Blood Glucose

Hyperglycemia (high blood glucose) means that your blood glucose level has risen and stayed well above normal or well above your goal range. There is no set number that defines hyperglycemia, because it can be different for different people. When your blood glucose level stays high, it means your diabetes is out of control.

CAUSES OF HYPERGLYCEMIA
High blood glucose can have many causes. Some of them are in your control, and others are not. From time to time, everyone with diabetes will experience hyperglycemia. Knowing the causes can help you to make a plan for taking care of high blood glucose right away.

Some of the causes include the following:

- Not taking your insulin or diabetes pills
- Getting sick
- Being stressed
- Eating too much
- Not getting your regular exercise

SYMPTOMS OF HYPERGLYCEMIA
You may have one or more of the following symptoms when your blood glucose level is high. Test your blood glucose if you:

- Are more thirsty than usual
- Are more hungry than usual
- Have to urinate a lot
- Have to get up more often at night to urinate
- Are more tired than usual
- Have problems with your vision
- Have dry, itchy skin
- Have an infection or cut that heals slowly

TREATING HYPERGLYCEMIA

- Take the right kind of medicine in the right amount at the right times.
- Eat the right kinds of foods in the right amounts at the right times.
- Exercise regularly or find ways to be more active in your daily life.

- Check and record your blood glucose every day. Your care team can help you decide how frequently and at what times to test.
- Keep your stress level under control.

Basic Sick Day Rules

1. Continue to take your insulin or diabetes medicine, unless your doctor has told you differently.
2. Test your blood glucose often—every 4 hours, or more often if told to do so.
3. Test your urine for ketones if you have type 1 diabetes.
4. If your blood glucose is less than 250 mg/dL, eat your normal amount of carbohydrate. If your blood glucose is more than 250 mg/dL, eat half of your normal amount of carbohydrate.
5. Drink lots of fluids—at least 8 cups a day.
6. Call your doctor if:

   Your blood glucose is greater than 250 mg/dL for 24 hours.

   You have ketones in your urine—moderate or high.

   You cannot keep down fluids and your temperature is higher than 101°F.

If you are unable to eat regular foods, try some soft solid or liquid foods. This list will help you choose the foods with the right amount of carbohydrates, calories, or exchanges for your meal plan. You may notice some foods on the list that you usually avoid. Remember that on a sick day, these take the place of your usual meals.

Food item	Carbohydrate content (g)	Approximate calories
Starch/bread exchanges		
1 slice bread	15	80
½ cup hot cereal	15	80
6 saltine crackers (2-inch squares)	15	80
4 soda crackers (2½ inch squares)	15	80
3 graham crackers (2½-inch squares)	15	80
½ cup ice cream (omit 2 fat exchanges)	15	170
1 cup broth soup (with noodles, rice)	15	80
1 cup soup, cream, reconstituted with water (omit 1 fat exchange)	15	125
½ cup tapioca	15	80

Food item	Carbohydrate content (g)	Approximate calories
Milk exchanges		
1 cup skim milk	12	90
1 cup low-fat milk	12	120
1 cup whole milk	12	150
1 cup yogurt (plain, skim milk)	12	90
1 cup yogurt (plain low-fat milk)	12	120
1 cup yogurt (plain, whole milk)	12	150
½ cup plain pudding	12	70
Simple carbohydrates		
½ cup ice milk (omit 1 fat exchange)	15	125
½ cup regular gelatin	15	80
¼ cup sherbet	15	80
4 oz regular carbonated beverages, cola type	15	55
Calorie-free foods		
Broth, beef or chicken[a]	—	—
Meat exchanges		
¾ cup low-fat cottage cheese	0	65
1 oz cheese	0	100
1 poached or soft-boiled egg	0	75
Vegetable exchanges		
½ cup tomato juice	5	25
½ cup vegetable juice	5	25
Fruit exchanges		
½ twin popsicle	10	40
Fruit juices (unsweetened)		
½ cup cranberry, grape, prune juice	15	60
½ cup canned fruit	15	60
½ cup cherry, grapefruit, orange, peach juice	15	60

[a] A good source of sodium, which may need to be replaced because of loss after vomiting and diarrhea.

Diet and Nutrition

Effects of Food on Blood Glucose

For a quick review, here's how diabetes and foods are related. Foods are the fuel or energy source for our bodies. Foods cannot be used for energy until the body changes them to a simple sugar called glucose. The blood carries glucose (blood sugar) to each cell in the body. Without glucose, cells do not have the energy to work.

Glucose needs help to get inside each cell. The helper that carries glucose inside the cells is called insulin, which is made by the pancreas, a body organ.

For a person with diabetes, food is changed into glucose just as in a person without diabetes, but either the body does not have enough insulin (type 1) or the glucose and insulin cannot get into the cell (type 2). Without insulin, glucose cannot get into the cell, so it builds up in the blood, causing high blood sugar, which may be harmful.

To bring the blood sugar down closer to a normal level, a special eating plan is always needed. Medication may also be prescribed to be used with the meal plan. To understand the eating plan, you need to know what makes up your foods.

NUTRIENTS

Foods contain nutrients and energy. The nutrients in food supply building blocks to the body. Food also contains energy that is measured in calories. Calories come from carbohydrates, proteins, fats, and alcohol.

CALORIES

Carbohydrates are the body's main source of energy. Carbohydrates are the starches in breads, cereals, and some vegetables and the sugars found in fruits and milk. The sugar that is in candy, cake, pie, jam, jelly, and honey is also a carbohydrate.

One hundred percent of carbohydrates that are digested break down to the energy packet glucose. This happens quickly.

Proteins are used to build and repair the body. Proteins are found in meats, fish, poultry, cheese, milk, eggs, and nuts. Proteins also break down to energy; 50% to 60% of the protein breaks down to glucose. This happens slowly.

Fats give a large number of calories or energy in a small bundle. Foods that contain fats are oils, margarine, butter, meat, and salad dressings. Use fats sparingly if you are trying to lose weight or if your blood fats are high. The body will store the fat and will break it down to smaller energy packets only in emergencies. So only 10% of fat will become blood glucose.

Managing Blood Sugar Through Your Diet

WHAT IS GOOD NUTRITION?

Good nutrition is eating a variety of different foods in combination to provide both necessary nutrients and good blood sugar control. No one food will supply all the nutrients your body needs.

Complex carbohydrates should be a big part of your meals and snacks. Carbohydrates come in two forms: simple and complex. Foods high in simple carbohydrates are cakes, pastries, candy, sugar, and honey. Simple carbohydrates raise your blood glucose quickly and to very high levels. These foods are also high in calories and fat and low in fiber and have few nutrients. Foods high in complex carbohydrates are vegetables, lentils and legumes, beans and peas, whole-grain unprocessed breads, cereals, rice, and pasta. Complex carbohydrates tend to slowly raise blood glucose and contain a variety of vitamins and minerals as well as fiber.

Good nutrition also means limiting your fat and cholesterol intake. Foods high in fats are gravies, sauces, salad dressings, fatty meats, and fried foods. High-fat foods have been linked to atherosclerosis, the fatty buildup inside the blood vessel walls. Atherosclerosis can contribute to heart disease and stroke. Also, foods high in fat are high in calories and can cause you to gain weight.

Some people may also be encouraged to limit sodium, which is found in large amounts in table salt and in highly processed foods.

Good Control Through Healthy Eating

Along with choosing the right foods, watch the amount of food you eat. For good diabetes control, you need to be consistent from day to day. Include carbohydrates at every meal. Plan your day to be sure you eat the right foods in the right amounts at about the same times every day.

A variety of foods that give a balance of carbohydrates and protein will help make sure there is glucose in your blood at the times your insulin is peaking (working the hardest) or during the times you are most active. Each meal should include a good source of carbohydrates and protein. This is the best balance for most people.

Samples of this type of balance include the following:

- Cereal and nonfat/lowfat milk
- A turkey sandwich
- Chicken or fish with pasta, rice, or potatoes

STEP 1: ANALYZE YOUR HABITS

For 3 days, record everything you eat, and note the time, place, and how you were feeling.

Do you eat when you are bored, upset, or under pressure?

Do you like to eat while reading or watching TV?

STEP 2: CHANGE YOUR BEHAVIOR
At Home

Eat at the kitchen or dining room table.

Eat sitting down.

Eat without reading or watching TV.

Keep tempting foods out of sight or reach.

Make tempting foods bothersome to prepare.

Have low-calorie foods ready to eat, in sight, and easy to reach.

Give other family members their own snack food cupboard.

When possible, stay out of the kitchen.

At Work

Do not eat at your desk.

Do not keep tempting food in your desk drawers.

Take prepackaged meals, snacks, and treats to work.

Use exercise instead of food for a break.

Carry no change for vending machines.

Eat a planned snack before leaving work.

Daily Food Management

Do not shop when hungry or tired.

Shop from a specific list—don't linger.

Don't buy your favorite varieties of high-calorie or hard-to-resist foods.

Prepare food when your control is highest.

Prepare lunches and snacks when another meal is being cooked, like dinner.

At Meals

Don't let serving bowls remain at the table.

Use smaller plates, bowls, and glasses.

Remove the plate as soon as you have finished eating.

If you are still hungry after a meal, make yourself wait 20 minutes before taking more.

Put utensil or food down between bites.

Cut food as it is needed.

Swallow your food before preparing the next bite.

Stop eating for a minute once or twice during the meal.

STEP 3: STAY ON TRACK

Take steps to avoid hunger, loneliness, depression, boredom, anger, and fatigue.

Look for your own "trigger situations," and identify personal strategies to change them.

Set short-term goals. When you reach your goal, reward yourself with a special nonfood item.

An Empty Shopping Basket and You

The oft-repeated trip to the supermarket can be a chore or an adventure—but it is always a necessity.

WHY SHOP SMART

Learning how to shop smart can help everyone make healthy food choices and get the most for their food dollar. Knowing this skill is key for the person with diabetes who must follow a food or meal plan.

THINK AHEAD—PLAN AHEAD

Planning and preparing meals is an art that must be developed. Like driving a car or riding a bicycle, it may look hard at first, but it's a skill that becomes easier with practice.

- Make a shopping list in advance to avoid return trips and forgotten items.
- Write a weekly menu of meals and snacks to be eaten at home.
- Take the weekly specials and seasonal items at your store into consideration.
- With menus as a guide, check the recipes you'll use (maybe there will be only one or two if you're off to work every day).
- Check the cupboard to make sure you have all the ingredients. While you're at it, make an inventory of food staples, cleaning supplies, and paper goods.
- Check through store coupons. Select coupons only for products you have planned to buy.

TIPS FOR SHOPPING

- If it's not on your list (and more so if it's not a healthy choice), then don't buy it!
- Shop when you're not hungry. This can help control impulse buying that can play havoc with healthful diets and your budget.
- Purchase fresh produce in small amounts.
- Seasonal fruits and vegetables are often better buys than out-of-season produce.
- Think about the quality you need.
- Buying in bulk isn't always the best choice—having more on hand may tempt you, or it may expire before you can use it all.

- Avoid tasting (because that's still eating) samples.
- Buy frozen and refrigerated foods last.
- Try shopping on the edges of the store—that's usually where you'll find the fruits, vegetables, meats, dairy products, whole-grain breads, etc. This will help you avoid most of the highly processed, high-fat foods.

Glycemic Index

The glycemic index compares the impact on blood sugar levels of the carbohydrate in foods with an equivalent amount of glucose. For example, if 1 g of glucose causes blood sugar levels to rise 10 points, 1 g of the carbohydrate found in a potato—or a serving of potato that contains 1 g of carbohydrate—will cause blood sugar levels to rise 7 or 8 points (70% to 79% of the 10-point rise caused by glucose).

To learn more information about the glycemic index, visit these web sites:

- *www. glycemicindex.com*
- *www.mendosa.com*

100%	80%–89%	70%–79%
Glucose	Cornflakes	Bread (whole meal)
	Carrots	Millet
	Parsnips	Rice (White)
	Potatoes (instant, mashed)	Weetabix
		Broad beans (fresh)
	Maltose	Potato (new)
	Honey	Swede

60%–69%	50%–59%	40%–49%
Bread (white)	Buckwheat	Spaghetti (whole meal)
Rice (brown)	Spaghetti (white)	Porridge oats
Muesli	Sweet corn	Potato (sweet)
Shredded Wheat	All-Bran	Beans (canned navy)
	Digestive biscuit	Peas (dried)
Ryvita	Oatmeal biscuit	
Water biscuits	"Rich Tea" biscuit	Oranges
Beetroot	Peas (frozen)	Orange juice
Bananas	Yam	
Raisins	Sucrose	
Mars Bars	Potato chips	

30%–39%	**20%–29%**	**10%–19%**
Butter beans	Kidney beans	Soya beans
Haricot	Lentils	Soya beans (canned)
Blackeye peas	Fructose	Peanuts
Chick peas		
Apples (Golden Delicious)		
Ice Cream		
Milk (skim)		
Milk (whole)		
Yogurt		
Tomato soup		

Sweeteners

Today, many products are available to sweeten our foods. Sweeteners are grouped into two categories: caloric and noncaloric. Some sweeteners have calories and carbohydrates; others have no calories or carbohydrates.

Sucrose (table sugar) is the most common caloric sweetener. People with diabetes used to be told to avoid or limit their intake of sucrose. The revised American Diabetes Association nutrition guidelines state that use of sucrose in meals or snacks does not harm blood glucose control.

The total carbohydrate content of a meal or snack does affect blood glucose levels. If you do use sucrose, you should include it in your meal plan with the help of your dietitian and doctor. It is still good advice to limit the use of foods with sucrose, as these foods are often high in carbohydrates and fat. If foods with sucrose are consumed, it is important to learn to adjust the intake of daily calories from other carbohydrate foods in your meal plan.

All caloric sweeteners contain about 120 cal/oz. Honey, fructose, and corn syrups are other common caloric sweeteners. These sweeteners offer no advantages over sucrose. Often, caloric sweeteners are "hidden" in processed foods. Ingredients that end with "ose" (such as lactose or sucrose) as well as invert sugar, raw sugar, and molasses are all examples of "hidden" caloric sweeteners. You should consider these ingredients when buying foods because they will increase the total carbohydrate content of foods.

Aspartame (Equal) and saccharin (Sweet 'n Low) are two noncaloric sweeteners on the market. Another low-calorie sweetener, acesulfame-K (Sweet One), is also available. It has 500 times the sweetening power of sugar, and, unlike aspartame and saccharine, acesulfame-K can be used in cooking and baking.

All of these sweeteners are safe for people with diabetes. Although they do not affect blood sugar levels, the Food and Drug Administration has measured their safety and set standards for "Acceptable Daily Intake" (ADI). The ADI is the amount of a food additive that can be safely consumed on a daily basis over a person's lifetime with no ill effects. When choosing foods with noncaloric sweeteners, it is important to read the label and be aware of other sources of carbohydrates and fats.

The chart below will help you choose the sweetener that will best control your blood sugar.

Sweeteners with calories

Sweetener	Calories	Carbo-hydrate	Comments
Sucrose *Examples:* beet sugar, brown sugar, cane sugar, confectioner's sugar, date sugar, invert sugar, raw sugar, saccharose sugar, succant, table sugar, turbinado, purinada	16 cal/tsp	4 g/tsp	Discuss the use of all caloric sweeteners with your dietitian.
Fructose *Examples:* fruit sugar, levulose	16 cal/tsp	4 g/tsp	Sweetness varies but may be almost twice as sweet as sucrose. Can be used in baking. Studies suggest that high intakes may increase cholesterol levels.
Glucose and glucose syrups *Examples:* corn sugar, corn syrup solids, dextrose, grape sugar, sorghum syrup, sugar cane syrup, unprocessed cane syrup	16 cal/tsp	4 g/tsp	Can be found in processed foods.
Sugar alcohols *Examples:* dulcitol, mannitol, sorbitol, xylitol	16 cal/tsp	4 g/tsp	May cause bloating, diarrhea. Does not usually cause a rapid or marked rise in blood sugar in well-controlled diabetes.
Miscellaneous foods *Examples:* carbo powder, honey, maple syrup, molasses, sweetened condensed milk	16 cal/tsp	4 g/tsp	None

Sweeteners with no or low calories

Sweetener	Calories	Carbohy-drate	Comments
Sucralose (Splenda)	None	Not absorbed	Can be used in baking and cooking. See *www.Splenda. com* or call 1-800-321-7254.
Acesulfame K (Sweet One, Sunette, Sweet 'N Safe)	4 cal/g	Very little carbohydrate and therefore little effect on blood glucose	Can be used in baking and cooking. For questions, call 1-800-544-8610.
Saccharin (Sweet 'N Low)	None	No carbohy-drate and therefore little effect on blood glucose	May have a bitter or metallic aftertaste in some liquids. Not suitable for baking and cooking.
Aspartame (Equal, Nutra Sweet)	None	No carbohy-drate and therefore little effect on blood glucose	Loses sweetness when exposed to heat. For questions, call 1-800-321-7254.
Whey Low when mixed	5 cal/tsp; with other carbohy-drates like oatmeal, calories decrease due to lack of absorption	1/g	Same sweetness as sugar; use and measure like sugar; brown sugar version (Gold), powder form and packets; it can be heated and acts like sugar; made from sucrose, whey, and fructose. Compete with each other for absorption site, so decreased or no calories if mixed with other carbohy-drates. Contact: *www.wheylow. com* or 1-888-639-8480.

Diabetes and Its Effect on Your Body

Diabetes and the Nervous System

WHAT ARE NERVES?

Nerves are special cells in the body that connect the brain with all other parts of the body. You could think of them as the electrical wiring of the body or the communications system. Nerves carry information to and from the brain to keep us safe and aware of our surroundings. For example, if you were walking barefoot and stepped on a sharp tack or nail, a signal would be sent very quickly up the nerves from your foot to the brain saying, "This is painful!" Your brain would very quickly send another signal down some other nerves, allowing you to quickly remove your foot from the tack.

HOW DOES DIABETES DAMAGE THE NERVES?

Because nerves are very long and thin, they are vulnerable to damage. Often the longest nerves, such as those that travel all the way to the feet, get damaged most easily. When blood glucose levels are too high, the chemistry in the nerve cells does not work properly. Nerves may also be damaged if their blood supply is reduced. Other conditions that have nothing to do with diabetes can also damage the nerves. These include vitamin deficiencies, lack of thyroid hormone, excessive alcohol intake, and smoking.

WHAT HAPPENS WHEN YOUR NERVES GET DAMAGED?

You may feel an unpleasant tingling or a sharp, burning sensation in your feet, which is often worse at night. Your feet may simply become numb so that it feels as if you are walking on cotton wool. Your feet or legs may also feel weaker than usual. If nerve damage affects your arms and hands, then pain, tingling, numbness, or weakness may be felt there also. Other symptoms may include dizziness when standing up, unsteadiness when walking, sweating, nausea and bloating after meals, and diarrhea. Men may develop erectile dysfunction if the nerves to the sex organs are damaged.

WHAT CAN I DO TO PREVENT NERVE DAMAGE?

To prevent nerve damage, take the steps needed to keep your blood glucose as near to normal as possible. In addition, don't drink much alcohol and don't use tobacco. Develop a healthy meal plan and stick to it.

CAN ANYTHING BE DONE IF I DEVELOP NERVE DAMAGE?

If you develop pain due to nerve damage, treatment is available, using medications. Often, the painful symptoms go away (or become much less severe) after a few weeks. Improving your blood glucose control may also help. Remember, if your feet have lost sensation, you need to take special care to protect them from damage.

Other symptoms, including bloating after meals, dizziness when standing up, and erectile dysfunction, can also be treated. If you have any unusual symptoms that you think might be caused by nerve damage, please talk to your doctor.

Diabetes and the Kidney

Diabetic nephropathy, also known as diabetic kidney disease, is a serious complication of diabetes mellitus. About 30% to 40% of patients with type 1 (insulin-dependent) diabetes will eventually develop kidney failure and require dialysis (or kidney transplantation). Only between 5% and 10% of patients with type 2 (non—insulin-dependent) diabetes develop kidney failure.

Diabetic nephropathy, like high blood pressure, has a long "silent" phase that lasts about 15 years. Currently, the only way to find out if kidney disease is present is to measure the amount of protein in the urine. Normally, there should be little, if any, protein present in the urine. Therefore, regular measurements should be part of the routine care of all patients with diabetes.

Once diabetic nephropathy is diagnosed, there are two treatments that we use to delay its progression. The most important is to control high blood pressure. Most, but not all, patients with diabetic kidney disease have high blood pressure. It is now clear that a class of blood pressure medication called ACE (angiotensin-converting enzyme) inhibitors not only lowers blood pressure, but also independently retards the progression of nephropathy.

The other treatment for diabetic nephropathy is a low-protein diet. Recent evidence suggests that a high-protein diet aggravates diabetic nephropathy. Therefore, many scientists believe that low-protein diets should be considered for patients with this disease. In fact, the American Diabetes Association recommends that *all* patients with diabetes should only eat 15% to 20% of their total calories as protein. Some hope that this lower-protein diet will help to prevent diabetic nephropathy.

Diabetes and the Eye

ARE EYE EXAMS NEEDED?

We are not able to predict who will be among the 3% to suffer eye problems. Therefore, it is essential that everyone with diabetes see an ophthalmologist (a medical doctor specially trained in eye disease) every 1 to 2 years. Annual eye exams are recommended for all patients with type 2 (non-insulin-dependent) diabetes.

However, any patient with diabetes who has eye discomfort should have an eye exam. Reporting changes in vision to your doctor and having your blood pressure checked can also help catch problems. The early detection and treatment of eye disease help protect your vision. The ophthalmologist will be looking for signs of diabetic retinopathy and for other problems such as cataracts and glaucoma.

WHAT IS RETINOPATHY?

Diabetic retinopathy is a deterioration of the small blood vessels that nourish the retina, a lining on the inside of the eye. The retina records visual images focused on it and changes them into electrical impulses that the brain can receive and understand.

Damage from retinopathy can occur before any symptoms, such as spots in the field of vision or vision loss from bleeding in the eye, begin. Some patients will experience a blurring of vision, which can be caused by swelling of the macula, the area near the center of the retina that is responsible for fine or reading vision.

An ophthalmologist can observe problems during a dilated eye exam with the help of special eye photography. Most often, though, patients will experience a blurring of vision, which is usually caused by swelling of the macula.

Current Treatment

Good success in treating retinopathy has been achieved with photocoagulation, a laser beam that can close off leaky blood vessels. This treatment is done by an ophthalmologist on an outpatient basis. Patients return home the same day.

WHAT ABOUT CATARACTS AND GLAUCOMA?

A cataract is a clouding of the lens of the eye, which interferes with the passage of light to the back of the eye.

As the cataract becomes cloudier, vision decreases. Cataracts can be treated by the surgical removal of the opaque lens. Although cataracts may not be more frequent in diabetic populations, they are four to six times more likely to develop at a younger age and progress more rapidly.

Glaucoma is an eye disease linked with increased pressure within the eye. It can damage the optic nerve and lead to impaired vision and blindness. The frequency of glaucoma is 5% in the diabetic population as compared with 2% in the population at large. Treatment ranges from simple eyedrops to surgery, depending on the type of glaucoma.

Care of the Feet

People with diabetes need to care for their feet on a daily basis. Diabetes often contributes to the development of decreased feeling or altered sensations (neuropathy) in the feet. Neuropathy can cause people with diabetes to lack the normal signals—discomfort or pain—which usually protect against foot problems. Diabetes can also be associated with the development of blockages in the blood supply to the feet. This is called atherosclerosis. Decreased circulation to the feet may make people with diabetes more prone to infections and slower healing of injuries.

The goal of daily foot care is to *prevent* any foot injury from occurring. If an injury does occur, bringing it to the prompt attention of your health care provider can help *prevent* a small problem from becoming a major concern.

1. Have your feet professionally examined at least once or twice a year.
2. Wash your feet daily, dry them well, and keep them dry. Always wear clean socks or stockings.
3. Inspect your feet daily, checking for redness, blisters, cuts or scratches, cracks between your toes, discoloration, or any other changes. Keep an eye on minor abrasions; keep them clean, and treat only with antiseptics recommended by your health care team. If you notice any infection, changes, or abnormalities, report these right away to your doctor or podiatrist. Because having diabetes may cause you to lose some feeling in your feet, regular inspection is essential. You can have an infection and not know it.
4. Prevent unnecessary cuts and irritations.
   - Do not wear rundown shoes or worn-out stockings.
   - Do not treat your own foot problems with sharp instruments or by probing into the corners of your toenails.
   - Do not walk barefoot, even at home.
5. Avoid burns, including excessive sunburns. Do not put your feet in hot water or add hot water to a bath without testing the water temperature. Generally, a bath should be between 85 and 90 °F. If you do not have a proper thermometer, test the water with your elbow. Avoid hot water bottles and heating pads. Hot

tubs and Jacuzzis are usually heated to >90 °F, so they should be used with extreme caution.

6. Avoid doing things that will restrict the blood flow to your feet, such as smoking, putting pressure on your legs, and exposing them to cold. Everyday activities such as sitting with your legs crossed or wearing round elastic garters or socks with tight elastic tops also can decrease the circulation to your feet.

7. Stay away from corn plasters or commercial corn or wart cures. These preparations are acidic and destroy tissue. Once you lose tissue, you have an opening in the skin, which *may* become infected.

8. When your toenails are trimmed, be sure they are cut or filed straight across. The length should be even with the end of the toe. Be sure to get assistance in trimming your nails, if you have any problem reaching them or seeing them clearly.

9. Wear shoes that fit your feet and the occasion. The widest part of the shoe should follow the natural outline of your foot and be snug but not tight. Wear special shoes or have your shoes adapted to your feet if you have a deformity. In general, shoes should support the heel and keep your foot in position. There should be about a ⅜- to ½-inch space beyond your longest toe when you stand. Shoes should also be roomy enough so that your toes do not hit or rub against the top of the shoe as you walk. The shoe upper should be soft and flexible. The lining should be smooth and free of ridges. Until you are used to new shoes, wear them for short periods and gradually lengthen the wearing time.

Diabetes and Your Well-Being

Stress and Diabetes

It would be perfectly normal for you to think that diabetes has just added one more (or much more) stress to your life. And stress can and will affect your diabetes control efforts. But stress can motivate us to do something new, to grow, to learn, and to make changes for the better.

Stress becomes harmful when there is no way to manage it, to make it work for you. Sometimes your personality makes it harder to manage stress. At other times, the situation creating the stress cannot be managed—or at least not right away or without help from others. Harmful stress is part of our lives. It is unrealistic to expect it can be totally eliminated.

Accepting that harmful stress is part of all of our worlds does not mean you should live in fear about how it affects your diabetes. Worrying about being out of control every time you fail to manage your stress perfectly will only create more stress.

SYMPTOMS OF STRESS

Each person responds differently to stress. Some common symptoms not already mentioned are dry mouth, heart beating faster, sweating, and heavier breathing. Some of the harmful responses to stress include the following:

- Hoping stress will go away
- Ignoring your feelings
- Trying to do it all yourself
- Thinking only about bad things
- Blaming yourself
- Expecting yourself to be perfect
- Expecting to be able to change everything
- Treating your body badly by smoking, drinking too much alcohol, undereating, or overeating

Stress that isn't controlled or managed can cause very uncomfortable feelings such as anger, frustration, depression, helplessness, fear, and guilt.

This just goes to show why setting good goals, building exercise into your daily life, eating a healthy, well-balanced diet, and getting support from family and friends are so important to good diabetes control.

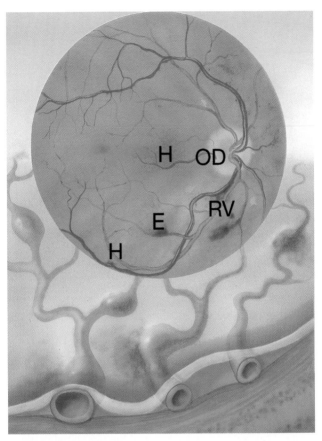

Diabetic retinopathy. Diabetes can cause changes in the eye that are usually not noted until significant bleeding occurs that interferes with your vision. This drawing shows the back of an eye, called the retina, with early changes from diabetes called nonproliferative diabetic retinopathy. Diabetic retinopathy is the deterioration of the small blood vessels that nourish the retina, causing a hemorrhage in the eye (H). Damage from this deterioration can occur before any symptoms such as spots or blurred vision become apparent. However, these early changes, as shown above, can be treated by a specialist in eye disease. Usually, laser therapy is employed. This is very effective in preventing blindness and is a good reason to see an eye doctor routinely, whether or not you are experiencing discomfort. E, exudates (small protein leaks); OD, optic disc (the nerve bringing images of light back to the brain); RV, retinal vein.

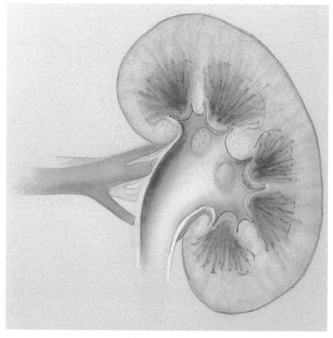

Diabetic nephropathy. Also called diabetic kidney disease, diabetic nephropathy is a serious complication of diabetes that can result in the need for kidney dialysis or transplantation. Diabetic kidney disease, and the high blood pressure that often accompanies it, have a long "silent" period of about 15 years, during which you may not experience any symptoms of the disease. To diagnose kidney disease during this period, your urine is checked for protein. Normally there is little to no protein in urine. Therefore, regular measurements can greatly increase your chances of early diagnosis and proper maintenance to control your high blood pressure and the progress of the disease with medication and a lower-protein diet.

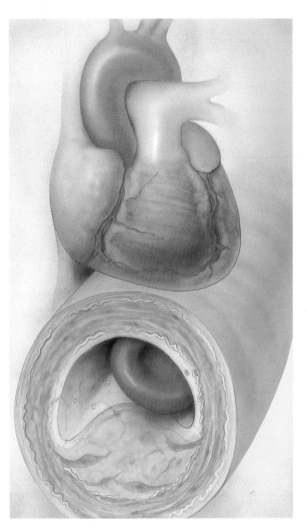

Atherosclerosis. Atherosclerosis is a blockage of blood vessels by material called plaque. A blockage, depending on its location, can result in loss of blood flow to your feet, as described in Fig. 4, or heart problems, as illustrated here. This is a cross-section of an artery. The plaque is the blockage at the bottom and consists of cholesterol, proteins, and connective tissues. Blood vessel disease is the number one long-term complication of diabetes and can result in heart attacks. Symptoms of heart disease can be much milder in diabetic persons than in others, so take very seriously any symptoms such as generalized weakness, mild difficulty breathing (being frequently "out of breath"), and "the sweats"—perspiring excessively. The best preventive measures are sticking to your diet plan and exercising regularly. Your doctor should help you design your diet and exercise regimens.

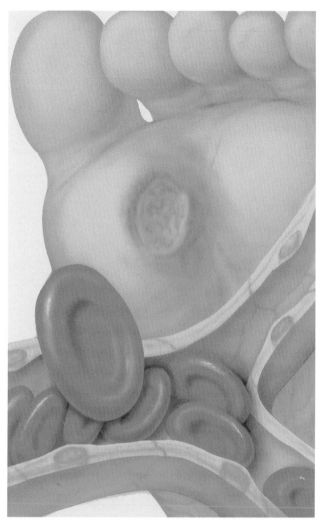

Neuropathic (loss of sensation) ulcers on a Charcot foot. Problems with feet are common in diabetes. The problems result from poor circulation and sometimes nerve damage that limits sensation on the surface of the skin. The feet are prone to ulcers in these circumstances. When the ulcers penetrate to the underlying bone, amputation is a risk. Careful attention to your feet is essential for your self-care regimen, and you should take seriously any loss of sensation to your feet and should report it to your doctor. Wash your feet daily and keep them dry. Check for redness, blisters, cuts or scratches, cracks between your toes, discoloration, and any other changes. Regular inspection is essential. You can have an infection or open sore and not know it.

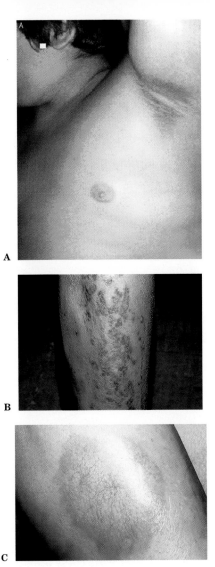

Diabetic skin problems. A: Acanthosis nigricans, a darkening of the skin found on the back of the neck and under the arms, indicates insulin resistance. Many people with type 2 diabetes develop this disorder. Acanthosis nigricans can be treated with weight loss, so check with your practitioner if you have this symptom. **B:** This is diabetic dermopathy, a term used for round brown or purple patches that appear on the shins. It occurs in up to 60% of diabetic patients. No treatment is required, as diabetic dermopathy is a common and benign symptom of diabetes. **C:** Necrobiosis lipoidica more often occurs in women than men and usually appears on the legs. The thin skin reveals blood vessels and other tissues that are not normally visible. This disorder may be of concern to the patient with diabetes, as what might be a small area of involvement can become quite large; however, this, like diabetic dermopathy, is a benign symptom of diabetes.

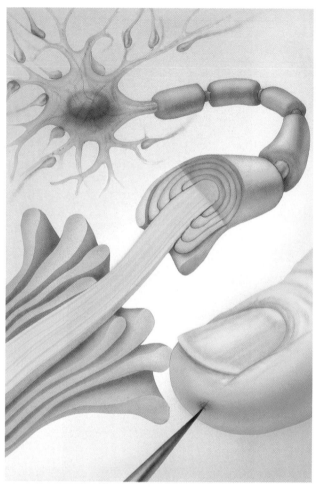

Nerve damage. Nerves are special cells in the body that connect the brain with all other parts of the body, transmitting information from your brain to keep your body safe and aware of its surroundings. Because nerves are long and thin, they are vulnerable to damage. When blood glucose levels are too high, as is the case in diabetes, nerves cannot function properly. You can prevent nerve damage by taking steps to keep your blood glucose as near to normal as possible with a healthy meal plan and a regular schedule for your medication. The symptoms of nerve damage may include a tingling, or "pins-and-needles," sensation in your feet, or your legs may begin to feel numb. You may also feel dizziness when standing up, unsteadiness when walking, or nausea. Consult your physician if you encounter any of these symptoms.

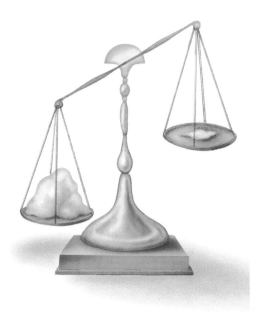

Low Blood Sugar (hypoglycemia):

causes: too much insulin

not enough food

unusual exercise

delayed meal

watch for: hunger

headache

irritability

personality change

excessive sweating

faintness

heart pounding

trembling

Hypoglycemia-

When blood sugar goes low-

for you, less than_____

treat with 15 grams of carbohydrate:

1/2-3/4 cup of non-diet soda drink

1/2 cup fruit drink or juice

2 tablespoons raisins

5 Lifesavers candies

1 cup milk

3 glucose tablets

follow by protein snack, such as:

1/2 meat sandwich

small pkg. cheese and crackers

Hypoglycemia chart. Low blood sugar (hypoglycemia) is a risk with treatment of diabetes. Listed are common symptoms and changes that can be seen with hypoglycemia as well as recommendations for prompt treatment. The best treatment is prevention: not skipping meals, checking blood sugar before and after exercise, and discussing with your health care provider any planned changes in your work or activity schedule and how this might require a change in your medication.

Page numbers followed by f *indicate a figure;* t *following a page number indicates tabular material.*

A

Acarbose
diabetes prevention, 107
dosing, 29t
mechanism of action, 34
side effects, 29t, 34
ACE inhibitors. *See*
Angiotensin-converting
enzyme (ACE)
inhibitors
Acromegaly, diabetes
association, 63
Advanced glycosylation end-
products (AGEs),
microvascular
complication role, 67
Aging
cognitive effects of
hyperglycemia, 100
diabetes epidemiology, 1
AGEs. *See* Advanced
glycosylation end-
products (AGEs)
Albuminuria
cardiovascular disease
management, 81
diabetic nephropathy, 70–72
screening
algorithm, 72f
etiologies of false-positive
tests, 72t
recommendations, 71–72
Alcohol
cardiovascular disease
prevention and risks,
84, 108
young male diabetic
concerns, 102–103
Aloe, diabetes management,
50
α-glucosidase inhibitors. *See*
Acarbose; miglitol
Alprostadil, erectile
dysfunction
management, 104–105

Amputation, prevention, 3
Angiotensin receptor blockers
(ARBs), benefits in
cardiovascular disease,
81
Angiotensin-converting
enzyme (ACE)
inhibitors
diabetic nephropathy
management, 73, 161
hypertension control
benefits in
cardiovascular disease,
81
ARBs. *See* Angiotensin
receptor blockers
(ARBs)
Aspirin, cardiovascular
disease prevention, 84
Atherosclerosis. *See*
Cardiovascular disease
Atypical diabetes
clinical features, 8
defect and genetics, 7t
Autonomic neuropathy
clinical presentation, 75
conduction disorders, 79
pre-exercise evaluation,
26
treatment, 75–76

B

β-blockers
diabetes induction, 65
hypertension control
benefits in
cardiovascular disease,
80–81
β-cell
insulin production loss by
time of diabetes
diagnosis, 28
islet cell transplants, 112
sulfonylurea effects on
function, 30

C

CAM. *See* Complementary and alternative medicine (CAM)

Carbohydrate
  counting, 16, 21
  diabetes type considerations in diet, 21–22
  sick day meals, 139–140
  snack content and hypoglycemia treatment, 129, 133, 135

Cardiovascular disease (CVD)
  aspirin therapy, 84
  atherosclerosis, 173f
  conduction disorders and outcomes, 79
  diabetic patient attitudes, 77
  glycemic control benefits, 79–80
  hypertension control benefits, 80–81
  ischemic episode presentation in diabetes, 78
  lifestyle modification in prevention, 83–84
  lipid lowering in prevention, 81–83
  mortality in diabetes, 77–78
  myocardial infarction
    angioplasty without stent placement outcomes, 78–79
    congestive heart failure incidence, 79
    mortality factors in diabetes, 78
  polycystic ovarian syndrome, 95–96
  pre-exercise evaluation, 25
  prevention, 3

Cataract, diabetes association, 69, 163–164

Chromium, diabetes management, 46–47

Cod liver oil, diabetes prevention in offspring, 108

Complementary and alternative medicine (CAM)
  aloe, 50
  chromium, 46–47
  definition, 46
  folic acid, 51–52
  γ-linolenic acid, 50
  garlic, 51
  ginkgo biloba, 50
  ginseng, 49–50
  magnesium, 48–49
  nicotinamide, 48
  practitioner knowledge of patient use, 52
  prevalence of use with diabetes, 46
  vanadium, 47–48
  vitamin E, 49

Continuous subcutaneous insulin infusion (CSII)
  implantable pump development, 111
  insulin requirements, 43
  principles, 42–43

CSII. *See* Continuous subcutaneous insulin infusion (CSII)

Cultural differences. *See* Ethnicity

Cushing's syndrome, diabetes association, 63

CVD. *See* Cardiovascular disease (CVD)

D

Depression
  identification and treatment, 91
  prevalence with diabetes, 86

Diabetes treatment targets, 119t

Diabetes type 1
  associated conditions, 8
  defect and genetics, 6t
  definition, 117
  insulin therapy
    continuous subcutaneous insulin infusion, 42–43
    correction insulin, 42, 43t
    dosing, 41t
    prandial and basal insulin replacement, 40, 42
    snack role, 42
  islet antibodies, 5, 7
  psychosocial issues
    comorbid conditions, 90
    complications, 89–90
    management routine, 88–89
    onset, 87
  puberty effects, 102

Diabetes type 1.5

clinical features, 10–11
defect and genetics, 7t
differential diagnosis, 11
treatment, 11
Diabetes type 2
    defect and genetics, 6t
    definition, 117
    diagnostic clues, 9
    insulin therapy
        basal insulin alone at
            bedtime, 43–44
        dosing, 41t
        indications for therapy, 43
        severe insulin deficiency
            patients, 44
        twice-daily injections, 44
    psychosocial issues
        comorbid conditions, 90
        complications, 89–90
        management routine,
            88–89
        onset, 87–88
Diabetes type 3
    clinical features, 11–12
    defect and genetics, 7t
Diabetic ketoacidosis (DKA)
    classification, 60
    clinical presentation, 60
    differential diagnosis, 60–61
    epidemiology, 59
    glucose levels at presentation,
        59
    laboratory findings, 60
    mortality, 59
    pregnancy, 99
    treatment
        complications, 62
        discharge, 62
        fluids, 61
        insulin, 61–62
        prevention of recurrence,
            62–63
Diabetic nephropathy
    albuminuria, 70–72
    epidemiology, 3, 69–70, 161
    pathogenesis and pathology,
        70
    pre-exercise evaluation, 25
    pregnancy, 98–99
    prevention, 3
    progression, 161
    retinopathy relationship, 71
    risk factors, 70–71
    screening
        algorithm, 72f

etiologies of false-positive
    tests, 72t
recommendations, 71–72
treatment, 73, 161
Diabetic neuropathy, 172f
    autonomic neuropathy, 26,
        75–76
    classification, 74t
    nerve damage mechanisms,
        159, 176f
    painful chronic sensorimotor
        neuropathy
        diagnosis, 74–75
        epidemiology, 73–74
        pathogenesis, 75
        treatment, 75
    pre-exercise evaluation, 26
    prevention, 160
    symptoms, 159
Diabetic retinopathy, 171f
    classification
        nonproliferative, 68
        proliferative, 68
    definition, 163
    eye examination, 163
    nephropathy relationship,
        71
    pre-exercise evaluation, 25
    pregnancy, 98
    prevalence, 68
    prevention, 68
    rapid glucose control
        exacerbation, 69
    screening, 68–69
    treatment, 69, 163
Diet. *See also* Medical nutrition
        therapy
    caloric intake requirements
        in adults, 23t
    glycemic index of foods,
        151–152
    good nutrition, 145
    grocery shopping tips,
        149–150
    lifestyle modification
        analysis of eating habits,
            147
        changing of behavior,
            147–148
        diabetes prevention,
            106–108
        obesity treatment, 23
        staying on track, 148
    nutrient types, 143–144
    sweeteners, 153–155

DKA. *See* Diabetic ketoacidosis
(DKA)

E
Eating disorders
identification and treatment,
91–92
prevalence with diabetes, 86
Economic impact, diabetes, 3
ED. *See* Erectile dysfunction
(ED)
Epidemiology, diabetes, 1–2
Erectile dysfunction (ED)
etiology, 103
evaluation, 103
prevalence, 103
treatment
alprostadil, 104–105
hypogonadism, 104
intracavernosal injections,
105
sildenafil, 104
Estrogen replacement therapy,
diabetics, 100
Ethnicity
diabetes epidemiology, 1–2
differences in views of
diabetes, 86–87
medical nutrition therapy
considerations, 22–23
Exercise
benefits, 25
blood glucose management by
diabetes type, 26–27
calories burned by physical
activity, 95, 96t
cardiovascular disease
prevention, 84
foot care, 26
lifestyle modification in
diabetes prevention,
106–107
pre-exercise evaluation
autonomic neuropathy, 26
cardiovascular disease, 25
diabetic nephropathy, 25
diabetic retinopathy, 25
peripheral neuropathy, 26
pregnancy, 98
prescription
recommendations, 16–17,
25
warm-up and cool-down, 26
Ezetimibe, blood lipid
modification, 83

F
Fat, medical nutrition therapy,
22
Folic acid, diabetes
management, 51–52
Foot care
exercise, 26
goals, 165
neuropathic ulcer on Charcot
foot, 174f
recommendations, 165–166

G
γ-linolenic acid (GLA), diabetes
management, 50
Garlic, diabetes management,
51
Gestational diabetes
complications and
management
diabetic ketoacidosis, 99
hypertension, 98
hypothyroidism, 99
nephropathy, 98–99
retinopathy, 98
definition, 117
epidemiology, 96
fetal surveillance, 99
labor and delivery, 99
management
diet, 98
exercise, 98
first trimester, 97
insulin therapy, 97
overview, 96–97
postpartum care, 100
prevention, 3
Ginkgo biloba, diabetes
management, 50
Ginseng, diabetes management,
49–50
GLA. *See* γ-linolenic acid (GLA)
Glaucoma, diabetes association,
69, 164
Glimepiride. *See* Sulfonylureas
Glipizide. *See* Sulfonylureas
Glucagonoma, diabetes
association, 64
Glucose
blood testing. *See* Glucose
tolerance test; self-blood
glucose monitoring
(SBGM)
metabolism, 143
sensors, development, 111

Glucose tolerance test, diabetes diagnosis and cut-off values, 2, 5
Glyburide. *See* Sulfonylureas
Glycemic index, foods, 151–152

H
Heat shock protein therapy, diabetes prevention, 108
Hemoglobin A1c
formation, 127
goal setting, 18
pregnancy targets, 97–98
testing, 127
HHS. *See* Hyperglycemic hyperosmolar syndrome (HHS)
HIV. *See* Human immunodeficiency virus (HIV)
Human immunodeficiency virus (HIV), medication induction of diabetes, 64
Hyperglycemia
causes, 137
cognitive effects in aging, 100
symptoms, 137
treatment, 137–138
Hyperglycemic hyperosmolar syndrome (HHS)
central nervous system manifestations, 53–54
epidemiology, 53
laboratory findings, 54, 55t
mortality, 53
precipitating factors, 56t
infection, 55
medications, 55, 57
metabolic illnesses, 55
treatment
anticoagulation, 58–59
fluid replacement, 57–58
insulin, 58
monitoring, 59
potassium replacement, 58
Hyperparathyroidism, diabetes association, 64
Hyperprolactinemia, diabetes association, 63
Hypertension, pregnancy, 98
Hyperthyroidism, diabetes association, 63
Hypoglycemia
affective disorders, 90
contributing factors, 66

definition, 65
epidemiology, 65
glucose cut-off values, 17
in-patient versus outpatient treatment, 66
management, 177f
diabetes type 1, 131
diabetes type 2, 129
middle of the night hypoglycemia, 135
snacks, 129, 133, 135
mortality, 65
symptoms, 17, 90, 131, 177f
treatment, 17
unawareness, 131
Hypogonadism, male, 104
Hypothyroidism, pregnancy, 99

I
Impaired glucose tolerance, definition, 118
Infection
hyperglycemic hyperosmolar syndrome precipitation, 55, 56t
prevention, 3
urinary tract infection in postmenopausal women, 100
Insulin
analog development, 110
challenges with standard insulins, 39–40
classification, 36–37
definitions of therapy, 37t
diabetes type 1 management
continuous subcutaneous insulin infusion, 42–43
correction insulin, 42, 43t
prandial and basal insulin replacement, 40, 42
snack role, 42
diabetes type 2 management
basal insulin alone at bedtime, 43–44
indications for therapy, 43
severe insulin deficiency patients, 44
twice-daily injections, 44
diabetic ketoacidosis management, 61–62
dosing recommendations by diabetes type, 41t

Insulin (contd.)
  hyperglycemic hyperosmolar
      syndrome management,
      58
  idealized absorption
      characteristics, 39f
  inhaled insulin development,
      110–111
  oral insulin development, 110
  pregnancy requirements, 97
  preparations, 38t
  production loss by time of
      diabetes diagnosis, 28
  programs for replacement, 37
  regimen of separate basal
      and prandial insulins, 40

K
Ketones
  home testing, 122–123
  monitoring, 17–18
  serum ketones in diabetic
      ketoacidosis, 60

L
LADA. See Latent autoimmune
      diabetes of adults (LADA)
Lancets, disposal, 125
Latent autoimmune diabetes of
      adults (LADA)
  clinical features, 10
  defect and genetics, 6t
  differential diagnosis, 11
  treatment, 11
Lipodystrophic diabetes
  clinical features, 12
  defect and genetics, 7t

M
Magnesium, diabetes
      management, 48–49
Maturity onset diabetes of the
      young (MODY)
  clinical features, 9–10
  defect and genetics, 6t
  glucokinase form, 10
  transcription factor form, 10
Medical nutrition therapy
  carbohydrate
      counting, 16, 21
    diabetes type
        considerations, 21–22
  cultural sensitivity, 22–23
  fat, 22
  goals, 20

  initial recommendations,
      15–16
  pregnancy, 98
  principles by patient type,
      20–21
  protein, 22
  weight management, 16
Menopause, diabetes
      considerations, 100
Meridia. See Sibutramine
Metformin
  benefits, 31–32
  combination therapy, 33
  diabetes prevention, 107
  dosing, 29t, 32–33
  mechanism of action, 31
  patient selection, 32
  polycystic ovarian syndrome
      management, 94–95
  side effects, 29t, 31–32
Miglitol
  dosing, 29t
  mechanism of action, 34
  side effects, 29t, 34
MODY. See Maturity onset
      diabetes of the young
      (MODY)
Myocardial infarction. See
      Cardiovascular disease
      (CVD)

N
Nateglinide
  dosing, 29t
  guidelines for use, 31
  side effects, 29t
Needles, disposal, 125
Nephropathy. See Diabetic
      nephropathy
Neuropathy. See Diabetic
      neuropathy
Niacin
  blood lipid modification,
      82–83
  diabetes induction, 64–65
Nicotinamide, diabetes
      management, 48
Nutrition. See Diet; Medical
      nutrition therapy

O
Obesity
  cardiovascular disease
      prevention, 83–84
  diabetes epidemiology, 2

lifestyle modification
  diabetes prevention,
    106–107
  treatment, 23
  pharmacologic intervention
    indications, 24
    orlistat, 24
    sibutramine, 24
  weight loss prescription, 23
Orlistat
  obesity management, 24
  side effects, 24

P
Pancreatic diabetes
  clinical features, 8–9
  defect and genetics, 7t
PCOS. *See* Polycystic ovarian
    syndrome (PCOS)
Peripheral neuropathy, pre-
    exercise evaluation, 26
Pheochromocytoma, diabetes
    association, 63
Physical activity. *See* Exercise
Physician visits, trends in
    diabetes, 4
Pioglitazone
  benefits, 33
  dosing, 34
  mechanism of action, 31
  side effects, 33–34
PKC. *See* Protein kinase C
    (PKC)
Polycystic ovarian syndrome
    (PCOS)
  diabetes and heart disease,
    95–96
  diagnosis, 94
  differential diagnosis, 94
  epidemiology, 93
  symptoms, 93–94
  treatment
    hirsutism, 95
    menses induction in
      adolescence, 94, 95
    weight loss, 95, 96t
Pregnancy. *See* Gestational
    diabetes
Protein
  medical nutrition therapy,
    22
  restriction in diabetic
    nephropathy, 73, 161
Protein kinase C (PKC)
  inhibitor development, 112

role in diabetic complications,
    68
Psychoeducational intervention,
    92
Puberty, diabetes effects, 102

R
Ramipril, diabetes prevention,
    107
Repaglinide
  dosing, 29t
  guidelines for use, 31
  side effects, 29t
Retinopathy. *See* Diabetic
    retinopathy
Rosiglitazone
  benefits, 33
  dosing, 29t, 34
  mechanism of action, 31
  side effects, 29t, 33–34

S
SBGM. *See* Self-blood glucose
    monitoring (SBGM)
Screening, diabetes, 1
Selective serotonin reuptake
    inhibitors (SSRIs),
    depression management
    in diabetes, 91
Self-blood glucose monitoring
    (SBGM)
  advantages over urine
    glucose, 13, 121
  disadvantages, 14
  discomfort minimization, 14
  frequency, 14
  glucose watch, 15
  goal setting, 18
  indications, 14
  meter selection and care, 122
  prick sites, 13
  reasons for testing, 121
  technology prospects
    computerized downloads,
      111
    smart insulin pens,
      111–112
  vision-limited patients, 14–15
Self-care barriers, 86–87
Sibutramine
  obesity management, 24
  side effects, 24
Sick day
  management, 18–19
  meals and rules, 139–140

Sildenafil
  efficacy, 104
  side effects, 104
Skin, diabetic complications
  acanthosis nigricans, 175f
  dermopathy, 175f
  necrobiosis lipoidica, 175f
Smoking, cardiovascular
      disease risks, 84, 108
Sorbitol, role in diabetic
      complications, 67
Spironolactone, hirsutism
      management in
      polycystic ovarian
      syndrome, 95
SSRIs. *See* Selective serotonin
      reuptake inhibitors
      (SSRIs)
Statins
  cardiovascular disease
      prevention, 81–83
  diabetes prevention, 107
Stress
  effects in diabetes, 169
  management, 169
  symptoms, 169
Sulfonylureas
  β-cell function effects, 30
  dosing

  glimepiride, 29t
  glipizide, 29t, 31
  glyburide, 29t
  mechanism of action, 30
  side effects, 29t, 30
Sweeteners
  acceptable daily intake, 153
  caloric sweetener types, 154
  classification, 153
  noncaloric sweetener types,
      155
Syringes, disposal, 125

T
Test strips, care, 122
Troglitazone, diabetes
      prevention, 107

V
Vanadium, diabetes
      management, 47–48
Viagra. *See* Sildenafil
Vitamin D, diabetes prevention,
      108
Vitamin E, diabetes
      management, 49

X
Xenical. *See* Orlistat